"My mom says no a lot, and it makes me mad sometimes but she always has a good reason even if I don't know it, sometimes I don't agree with the reason, but she still lets me state my opinion and she considers it, and then she says no... but I love her a lot –"

~Elora (11 years old – Betsy's Daughter)

"Do everything in moderation", she said. This was one thing my mom told me early on and whenever I feel myself going too far or too guilty or too much of anything I always hear that in the back of my head."

~ Erica (Debbie's grown up daughter)

"My mom sometimes works too much, but I love it when she throws the football, even if she's not very good at it."

~Max (8 years old – Betsy's Son)

"One of my favorite memories growing up was learning to read. Eventually my mom would read a chapter aloud and then I would. This might be why I love sharing stories to this day."

~Adam, Debbie's grown-up son

It Came Out of my Vagina! *Now What?!*

An Honest (like really honest) Guide to Parenting

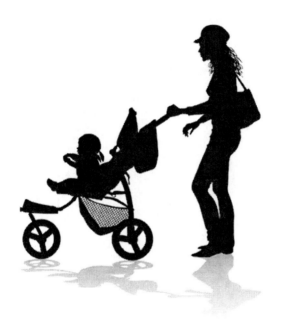

By Betsy Chasse and

Debbie Spector Weisman

Copyright 2015 to Betsy Chasse and Debbie Spector Weisman

www.betsychasse.net www.thedreamcoach.net

All rights reserved. Printed in the United States of America & the UK. No part of this book may be used or reproduced in any manner whatsoever without written permission, except in the case of brief quotations embodied in critical articles or reviews.

Although every effort has been made to ensure that the information in this book is correct at the time of going to press, the authors have written from their own view point and therefore all information is a personal opinion. The author and publisher assume no liability to any party as a result of the contents of this book.

The stories in this book are based on the authors' own personal experiences of their parenting journey and the outcomes of other people journeys that they may have witnessed. Although we have made every reasonable attempt to achieve complete accuracy in the content of this book, we assume no responsibility for errors or omissions in the information.

These stories have been shared as examples and inspiration only and we cannot guarantee you will achieve the same results in your own journey. If you choose to use this information in your own parenting you do so at your own risk. The methods and outcomes in this book are a result of observations by the author in their own life and the lives of their children. The information is not shared in a professional capacity and does not constitute as professional advice for your own situation. Please consult an expert if that is what you require.

How you choose to use the information in this book is completely your own responsibility and is done at your own risk. No responsibility will be taken for implications of safety while caring for your children. Your child, or whichever child is in your care at the time of while following the guidelines in this book is your own responsibility to be safe not of the publisher or authors.

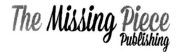

The Missing Piece Publishing

Seathorne Walk

Bridlington

East Yorkshire, YO16 7QP

England

For information visit www.themissingpiecepublishing.com

Book & Cover Design by Jennifer Insignares www.yourdesignsbyjen.com

Proof Reader : Amanda Horan www.gobookyourself.info

Book Layout: Kate Gardner www.the-missing-piece.net

Formatting: Bojan Kratofil https://www.facebook.com/bojan.kratofil

ISBN: 978-1-5136-0675-0

Praise from Real Moms

"Finally a parenting book that pulls no punches, tells it like it is, bursts your bubble and somehow makes you want to do it anyway! This is life and we are all merely human, so superhero parenting books only serve to make most people feel inadequate. No worries of that happening here. With each page you will congratulate yourself that your child is still alive and likely, will grow into an awesome adult." -Adryenn Ashley, Mom of a Son, tv host, award winning best-selling author of Every Single Girl's Guide to Her Future Husband's Last Divorce.

"Being a mom is both exhilarating and exhausting and this book reminded me to laugh and to relax, it's all going to work out." -- Candace Mollareza, Mom to a Daughter and a Son

"This book is honest, raw and downright hilarious. I wish I had read this book when I was a new mom, I certainly would have felt a whole lot better about my parenting skills and probably would have saved me from myself a few times!" -Stephanie Urbina Jones, Mom to a Daughter, #1 Billboard Artist #1 Songwriter, CEO Texicana Entertainer.

This book is awesome! The read truth on being a mom, it made me realize I am an awesome mom!" – Laura Cassidy Dreary Mom to a Daughter

"Being a single mom, heck being a mom is sometimes traumatizing, but always rewarding, this book helps you get through the hard parts so you can enjoy the fun ones" -Trish Miner Taylor Mom to a Son

"You can always count on Betsy to be boldly honest and always funny! And she definitely delivered both with this laugh-filled book overflowing with happy reminders that moms are amazing and loved!" – Marsh Engle – Author, Speaker and mom to two Sons

"You've heard it before, being a mom is the hardest and most rewarding experience you'll ever have, but you have never heard it like this, be ready to laugh, cry and remember you're not alone on this wild mommy ride" -Cindy Ertman, Author, Speaker mom to

Table of Contents

Prologue 1

Preface 8

Introduction 13

Chapter 1: The Birth Plan – LOL! 18

Chapter 2: Bringing Home Baby 32

Chapter 3: Surviving Other Family Members 47

Chapter 4: Feeding Facts and Myths 58

Chapter 5: What?! You Didn't Pre-register for Daycare the Moment You Got Pregnant? 73

Chapter 6: Managing Their Meltdowns…and Yours 89

Chapter 7: Tales from the Potty Training and Sleep Wars 103

Chapter 8: Baby Envy 118

Chapter 9: Mom Envy 128

Chapter 10: Teamwork, or How to Survive Being a Sports Mom 140

Chapter 11: Wait, This Isn't My Sweet, Obedient Child! What Happens When Your Kids Hit the Pre-Teen Years and the Hormones Start Kicking In 150

Chapter 12: The Battle of the Bulge…or Yes, You Can Get That Bikini Body Back 164

Chapter 13: What to Do with All Those Pictures? 178

Chapter 14: Yes, It's Time to Have Sex 188

Chapter 15: How to Avoid Mommy Guilt 197

Chapter 16: Letting Go 202

Chapter 17: The Single Mom 211

Chapter 18: Milestones You'd Rather Not Have... But Probably Will Anyway 220

Chapter 19: Other Mommies Weigh In: Opinions are like Vagina's every lady has one and we'd like to share some thoughts from other Mommies about their parenting experiences. 234

Chapter 20: The Final Word On Being a Mom 317

About the Authors 322

Contributing Authors 324

Prologue

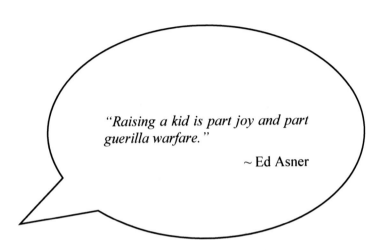

"Raising a kid is part joy and part guerilla warfare."
~ Ed Asner

There's a certain irony to Betsy asking me, a confirmed non-mother in the biological sense, to write the prologue to this book. But then, from what I've observed over the years, parenting is an essentially ironic condition, so it makes sense.

I mean come on. You eagerly, even desperately, desire a baby for *years*, only to discover the arrival of your little bundle of joy means at least a decade of sleep deprivation, the end of private phone conversations, uninterrupted sex, all possible hope of alone time, long martini lunches and walks on the beach with friends unencumbered by beach bags, toys, and baggies filled with peanut butter and sand.

But that's okay. It's nothing compared to the reward of being emotionally lacerated as the kids you'd willingly lay down your life for declare their eternal hatred over an endless array of important issues ... like not letting them play in the street or wear makeup at age eight, or date at ten or get multiple tongue piercings over summer vacation.

The whole child-rearing dynamic reminds me of the time I was in South Africa on a (camera) safari out in the bushveldt and came across a large troop of baboons. I was astonished at the mother/child interactions, which were clearly highly physical, love/hate relationships.

I remember watching one baby baboon. She kept bugging her mother as the troop grazed across the veldt, jumping on her, pulling her fur, distracting her from her food then running off, over and over again.

Fun right?

By Betsy Chasse and Debbie Spector Weisman

Finally, momma baboon lost it. She grabbed her darling baby on the next pass, screamed at her then hurled her about eight feet away through the air. Tumbling into the bushes and dirt, the baby picked herself up and ran, shrieking, to another large female, hurtling into her long hairy arms, seeking comfort.

The big female obliged, hugged her and started carrying her. Seeing this, momma baboon went into a jealous rage, ran over to the other female, knocked her in the head, plucked her baby from her grip and ran off with the infant.

I was deeply impressed. Unlike humans, baboon mothers are not uncertain or easily guilted. They don't read parenting books. They don't worry about scarring their children for life. They're simply really really clear about what works and what doesn't.

Humans, apparently, don't have it so easy.

I'm not sure if Betsy asked me to write this introduction for the clarity (and implied wisdom) of my more removed perspective or whether she simply couldn't get somebody more famous to provide this service. Either way you're stuck with an introduction to a parenting book that talks about baboons and the Indian

It Came Out of my Vagina! Now What?!

Goddess Shiva. I swear this Goddess is depicted as having eight arms because of all the things a typical adult human female has to juggle in her life. Which finally brings me around to Betsy and Debbie.

Betsy is a single mother of two, a filmmaker, author, college-level teacher, media consultant, ex-wife, lover and friend, she's one of the most talented human beings I've ever met and also (no surprise) one of the busiest.

For over a decade I've watched her from my diaper-less, thoroughly well-rested ivory tower and come to the conclusion that Betsy is also one of the best moms I've ever seen. (Which, now that I think about it, might be the reason she asked me to write this. Nothing like a good review!)

So why do I think she's a good mom? Well, she's clear with them. She communicates with them and treats them like intelligent beings. She is also baboon-level clear that her children come first.

Everything else fits in around them and somehow it all gets done. I think she has ten arms not just eight. She's also not perfect. (Whatever the hell *that* is.) I've seen her lose it and yell at her kids.

By Betsy Chasse and Debbie Spector Weisman

I've watched her discipline them and seen the fur fly. And I've listened to her talk about her guilt over such things over many a glass of wine at night.

Debbie I don't know so well. But she's successfully raised two children to adulthood and neither one of them has turned out to be an axe murderer. Which, I swear sometimes, is the best any parent can legitimately hope for. And having read this book I know she's got a level head and a great sense of humor about the whole thing.

Bottom line both Betsy and Debbie have successfully struggled for, and gained balance and perspective—something every parent must do—between the urge to play out their simian genetic heritage and throw their kid into the bushes (or maybe the ice cream freezer in the grocery store) in frustration and becoming a guilt-ridden doormat for the abuse children inevitably and unconsciously end up heaping on their parents over the years.

Sure. It's satisfying to know that when your kids finally have kids of their own they'll look back on their own upbringing with new eyes, and you'll get a phone call someday and have a great conversation, laughing over the whole thing. But thirty years is a long time to wait for a little compassion from ungrateful offspring.

Which is why Betsy and Debbie have written this book. To help you help give yourself a break, get some perspective, and, best of all, laugh. Because laughter is one of the only things that gets us through life—and one of the main things that separates us from the baboons.

~ Cate Montana

Author – Finding Venus, The E Word, Ego, Enlightenment and other Essentials

Olympia, Washington

Betsy: I actually asked Cate to write this because of the baboon story, it simultaneously made me laugh and cringe, having felt like that mother baboon on more than one occasion. Except I think that baboon has a better butt than I do. I also asked her because as a woman and friend she's an honest and great sounding board, mother or not. My first tip in this book is, don't lose your childless

By Betsy Chasse and Debbie Spector Weisman

friends just because they don't have kids, and you think they won't understand you. Trust me, you're going to want to have some grown up conversations which don't revolve around your kids poop schedule. Stay connected to the outside world; it will help remind you that there is a life beyond your kids and in doing so, you'll be a better mom.

Preface

Here's what most people will never tell you about becoming a parent. It sucks. Once that baby pops out, your life, as you know it, is over. No more sleep, no more peeing by yourself, no more perky tits, and say bye-bye to that bikini-worthy tummy. And that's the truth…well okay, maybe not really the whole truth.

Certainly it's closer to the truth than what you're probably imagining—bliss filled nights gazing lovingly at your sweetly sleeping child, fun-filled days at the park endlessly swinging your perfectly-behaved daughter or son while singing the songs your mother sang to you. Seriously, you need to lower your expectations because it's more likely that baby is going to scream bloody murder when you try to get s/he to sleep. And you're going to have to learn some really mean wrestling moves in order to commandeer a swing at the park from another mom who's had more practice than you.

Betsy: About a month into parenting my first child I realized that I had been had, that there must be some secret oath taken by other mommies to hide the truth of how hard parenting actually is, just to trick me into popping out a baby so I too could suffer like them. All those adorable baby pictures, all that laughter and tears of joy were a ruse. I could now see that jubilant laughter was just a means to hide the gagging they were doing from smelling all the vomit stains they were continually cleaning off the back seats of their cars and themselves.

But all kidding aside – wait I'm not actually kidding, well okay I'll admit it--I love my children more than I have loved anyone or anything in this world, even chocolate. But I wish someone had been a little more honest with me from the get go. I do think people mean well, suggesting what books to read and what baby things to buy, but the instead of empowering me to be the most confident mom I could be, all that non-solicited advice ended up making me feel like a failure. From the moment that stick and my fingers were drenched with that baby infused urine I was in a panic, because it's one thing to screw up Martha Stewart's latest do-it-yourself napkin rings, but there isn't enough Gorilla Glue or glitter to fix a real life do-it-yourself baby. That shit is for real and forever.

It Came Out of my Vagina! Now What?!

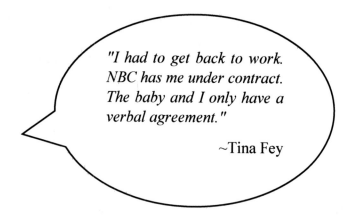

"I had to get back to work. NBC has me under contract. The baby and I only have a verbal agreement."

~Tina Fey

Debbie: As the youngest of three girls and the youngest child in my parents' circle of friends, I was never exposed to babies growing up. My image of babies was the lovely cooing kids I saw on television, those picture-perfect babies in those picture-perfect images of homes in my mom's magazines, and, of course, my own real-life experience changing and re-changing the diaper on my Betsy Wetsy doll. Honestly, I believed a real life baby couldn't be much different from that doll. I mean, she cried and all, with real tears coming out of those big blue eyes, and she looked so cute in all those pretty clothes I had for her.

Okay, so the tears were water and a plastic doll never squirmed and played the I-dare-you-to-get-that-diaper-on-me game on a

By Betsy Chasse and Debbie Spector Weisman

daily basis. Yes, I, too, came to parenting a bit on the naïve side. I believed that I could feed and diaper my daughter, put her in an infant seat, and then do whatever I pleased until the next regularly scheduled feed and change cycle. Nobody ever bothered to tell me differently.

Parenting was a giant wake-up call for me.

Neither of us hold degrees in early childhood development. What we are is two down-to-earth moms, one with two kids (7 and 11) and another with two grown kids and a grandbaby—both of whom want to tell it like it is (at least from our experience. We'll tell you what those other mommies won't.)

Our hope is you'll laugh at us and with us. Even more, we hope you'll learn to chill out and relax and *enjoy* parenting more. Along the way you might even pick up a few tips on how to quickly remove baby poop stains from satin nightgowns (or cotton which is more likely). Or that eating baby food isn't an awesome way to lose the baby weight. We both do prescribe loosely to the concept of conscious parenting, which is essentially connecting with your kids, listening to them, and offering them opportunities to learn emotional intelligence and to trust in their own instincts and intuition. But again, we aren't experts in that either as you're about to find out when you read this book.

Truth is, there is no ultimate child-rearing instruction manual. We made a conscious effort in this book to deal with the most common parenting issues. Therefore, you won't get any advice here on such serious topics as autism, childhood diseases, gun violence in school, child abuse, vaccines, gangs and the like. There are plenty of other books that deal with these very important issues. But getting real about having kids—having real moms talk about real parenting in down and dirty terms while rooting for you every step of the way—is probably a great start.

By Betsy Chasse and Debbie Spector Weisman

Introduction

> *I have a 25 and 35 year old! YES, I'm that old (64) and a lot more fun than thirty five years ago, when the first one was born. Laughter with a dash of crazy slathered on heavily works well. We all think we're terrible parents at some point, yet somehow they turn out better than us. Miracles happen.*
>
> *Parenthood is the greatest of gurus. Humbling to the core and they learn what they see and by your actions not our words. Now, that's pressure to stand up and fly high."*
>
> ~ Wendy Keown mom of two.

Betsy: Type in Parenting books in the search bar on Amazon and you'll find over 200,000 titles all ready to tell you the "right" way to parent: how to get your baby to sleep, how to make them geniuses, when they should be doing what and what they shouldn't be doing, how to be a good mom and basically to make you feel like you're a horrible, terrible and inadequate parent. You either read these books while you were pregnant and had those weird

It Came Out of my Vagina! Now What?!

pregnancy dreams about how your child turns into the evil spawn of Satan and eats you all because you fed them the wrong baby food, or a daemon because didn't play the right music during pregnancy, causing you to drive all the way to Walmart at 2 am to buy the baby genius CDs. Might as well start early... right? Or your baby is born and older and you're following the Dr. Sears schedule and when your baby doesn't crawl on the date you've circled in your calendar you go into sheer panic, calling every pediatrician, your mom, your mom's friends, balling your eyes out because your baby is a slow learner. You're lost, should they sleep on their tummy or their back, in the crib or in your bed, cloth or disposable diapers, to breast feed or not... OY. It's exhausting, overwhelming and stressful! Not to mention all the unsolicited parenting advice you're getting from everyone...and I do mean everyone, including the lady in line at the grocery store. Well we hope to counter all that with a few laughs, some nods of agreement "I've been there" and a message to just relax, listen to your heart and to the heart of your child and everything will be just fine. At least that's what I'm going to go with. There isn't a week that goes by where I don't

By Betsy Chasse and Debbie Spector Weisman

wake up wondering if I'm doing it all wrong, when one of my kids isn't happy with me or I look at them and wonder who are these aliens and what have they done with my sweet adorable children?!

Debbie: As you may be able to tell from this introduction, most of the chapters are going to be divided into two, one part from Betsy and one part from me. We flipped a coin about who would go first.

I suffer from IWIKTWIKN. I don't know if that's a real acronym or not, but it should be. Simply put it means "I wish I knew then what I know now". This holds true in many areas of my life, but none as important as my children.

I'm a Baby Boomer and when I was young we really thought we were hot shit and knew all the answers to everything. We didn't need to learn anything from our parents because they were old, unhip and tone deaf to the modern ways of the world. We were writing new rules, new ways of being, and one of those rules was that anything goes. *Take it easy, we can work it out* were popular song lyrics and philosophical paths to follow. Want a baby?

It Came Out of my Vagina! Now What?!

Simple. Give birth and *give peace a chance*. It all works out in the end. *All you need is love.*

When I was pregnant it might as well have been the dark ages as far as baby advice went. Sure there was the big bible that everybody read, Dr. Spock's *Baby and Child Care* and some good books about child development, but most of those were clinical in nature and spoke about the most idyllic situations. I lived in a very conventional suburb and came from a very traditional family, so there was no New Age enlightenment for me. There was no internet, no websites or blogs about parenting, no Facebook pages where new parents could go for support. There was this new idea floating about at the time, support groups called *Mommy and Me*, and those were considered groundbreaking since there was nothing like that for my mother when I was a baby. Progress!

What you have here is the book I wished I had when I was a young, naïve mother who at times felt completely out of her element…and, more often than I care to admit, out of my mind. Yes, I've made my share of mistakes in raising them, thus my

By Betsy Chasse and Debbie Spector Weisman

IWIKTWIKN lament. I'm a mother who has seen successes and failures, breakthroughs and breakdowns, victories and defeats and is still standing tall. Spoiler alert. I have raised a son and daughter to adulthood and they've not only survived, they've thrived. They didn't grow up to be Indigo Children or 21st Century Einsteins. But that's okay. Both are highly capable responsible members of our society and I love them unconditionally and forever. While I can't take total credit for their development, at least I can say that I haven't screwed them up. In this day and age, that's something for which to be thankful. If you go by the saying of, "What doesn't kill you makes you stronger", then I guess that makes my parenting skills a success.

So, dear reader, this book is dedicated to you. Do as I say and not as I did and you'll be a wonderful parent to your little loved ones.

Chapter 1
The Birth Plan – LOL!

> "I was so tired that I begged the doctor to get the "salad tongs" to pull her out... I may have been a little delirious... They refused to comply saying she'd be born with a cone head."
>
> ~ Mesa Fama, Filmmaker mom of 2

Betsy: I've never been a patient person, so sitting with my pants down, holding a pee-drenched stick waiting to find out if my world will be forever altered by a beautiful bundle of joy was probably the most excruciating sixty seconds I've ever endured. I sat and stared at the stick as the hue of pink slowly crept in.

By Betsy Chasse and Debbie Spector Weisman

If you've ever taken a pregnancy test, you know it starts out looking negative with the sad little (–) sign and then suddenly in pops another and you've got a baby on the way!

Woohoo— you did it! After the excitement wears off, you've shared the happy news and everyone is thrilled for you (oh, and suddenly a parenting expert), reality sets in. Luckily for me, in those early months as my body evolved into its new state, I didn't have morning sickness. I did miss my morning smoke and my evening glass of vino, but for the first few months I was in pregnancy bliss. That was, until I started to grow; I mean like *really* grow. All of my body-conscious buttons were being pushed and I spent a small fortune keeping Pea in the Pod in business. This wasn't just any pea in my pod, this was some sort of ginormous being growing in me.

I lived in a community that was all about all natural home births and all I could think about was how in the hell this gargantuan creature was going to come out of me. Every mommy I encountered wanted to share her birth story (okay I admit it, I'm guilty of this too). It's a badge of honor; when you pop a human the size of watermelon out of your Vagina, you're going to want to brag about it too. But with each triumphant "push!" story I began to feel more and more stressed out. I eventually decided to go with the flow. I'd have my own home birth, with my own hand-picked midwife who urged me to write my own birth plan. I ordered the birthing tub, created my play list, went to the Lamaze classes and grew and grew…and grew. As the birth date approached, my nesting instinct took over. I had either registered for or bought every possible baby gadget a mommy could want. The nursery was ready, the house was cleaner than it had ever been, and I was ready.

I was amazed at the little wheel my midwife used to calculate the exact date my baby would arrive in this world. I circled that date on my calendar, cleared my schedule and manically planned my every step for the days leading up to the birth and the week after. In hindsight, I realize how futile this was. It was simply an attempt to hold on to some control of an event that I had no control over at all.

It's a funny thing, those due dates. Seriously, most babies never get the memo, my baby included. So my first piece of advice

By Betsy Chasse and Debbie Spector Weisman

to you is this: Chill. That baby will come when it's damn good and ready!

That lack of control became evident the moment I went into labor. I had spent the evening in Seattle, and it was nearing midnight when, after a two-hour drive, I was finally heading down my long driveway lovingly referred to as the plains of Mordor. Along the way I felt something stirring down there. Thankfully, my water waited until I got in the house and then suddenly…gush!

I awoke my sleeping husband and we leapt into action. Timing contractions, calling the midwife, filling the birthing tub. About three hours later my midwife arrived and for the next 18 hours I was in labor. Yep, 18 hours and *still* no baby. So much for my "have-her-out-in-five–hours" plan. This baby girl was having none of that!

We were in the tub, out of the tub, in a chair, in the bathroom (all places I never expected I would be giving birth, except the tub—it was all about the tub). But truth be told I hated that tub. For god's sake, seriously, whose idea was it for me to squat in a lukewarm kiddie pool, gushing amniotic fluid and pushing like my

It Came Out of my Vagina! Now What?!

life depended on it?! Oh wait, it was my idea. I had watched the videos, read all the books and listened to all those mommies share their fairy-tale birth experiences in water, and somehow I must have screwed something up. Did I buy the wrong candles? Should I have purchased the pool with the turtles on it instead of the goldfish? Maybe it was the music. Yes, that was it, the music. Clearly I should have gone with Mozart instead of "It's the end of the world as we know it".

Well, whatever it was, my birth plan had gone to hell in a kiddie pool with goldfish on it.

Here's the thing. Women forget about the pain, the doubt, the fear and the absolute horror of giving birth mere seconds after that baby is out and in their arms. So often the birth stories you hear may joke about the pain, but no one ever lets you in on the secret that giving birth hurts like hell! Even as I write this I have to work to remember how hard it was. Our brains are wired that way; otherwise who the hell would do it again?

After it was clear this baby was not coming out, it was decided I should go to the hospital. I was surrounded by people who for

By Betsy Chasse and Debbie Spector Weisman

months told me awful stories about hospitals, and there I went, this time with my husband and midwife, back down the plains of Mordor. Only this time I was having full blown contractions while on a 45-minute drive to the nearest hospital. Yay me! Yes, this is exactly how I planned to have my baby— on the side of the freeway in the wee hours of the morning. Finally, I was wheeled in through the emergency room doors, plugged in and my labor stopped. Yep, the hospital stopped my labor, only to restart it a few hours later (I learned after the fact that I inconveniently showed up in the midst of a shift change. The gall of me and my baby!)

Forty hours after my labor began I was told I needed a C-section. The sad but honest truth is that in that moment they could have told me I was getting a lobotomy and I wouldn't have cared— I just wanted this baby out. I actually recall screaming that as I was hanging from a bar on a hospital gurney attempting one last time to push that stubborn little pea out of my pod.

Since I had been given an epidural, I was able to stay awake during the C-section, and I have to tell you, it was awesome. Well,

It Came Out of my Vagina! Now What?!

at least the drugs were awesome and finally she was out; I instantly forgot about everything else – thanks brain!

It wasn't until a few hours later, when the drugs wore off and I attempted to forgo the pain meds so as not to affect my breast milk did the memories flood back in: the sweat, the tears, and the excruciating pain. But not for long. See—after you have a C-section, the most important thing on your mind is, *"Can I poop without my gut exploding?"* The answer, thankfully, was yes, and despite my concerns, my gut didn't spill out onto the floor.

Now I have shared my birth story, here's what you should do with it. Smile and say thank you—and then forget everything I just said. Your birth is your birth. It will happen as it happens. Trust in your own abilities to listen to your body and your baby, find a midwife or OBGYN you love and listen to them.

> *"Motherhood is tough. If you just want a wonderful little creature to love, you can get a puppy."*
>
> -Barbara Walters

By Betsy Chasse and Debbie Spector Weisman

Debbie: Betsy is right. Your birth is going to be whatever it is, and whatever is it will most likely *not* be what you're expecting. That's how it was with me. It was a different time and a different generation. So many things that are commonplace now, like midwives and home births, were alien concepts then. The idea of having husbands in the delivery room was pretty much standard practice where we lived, but there were still some backward sections of the country where people were just coming on board.

There was no doubt in my mind I was having a hospital birth, and with my living in Los Angeles and being Jewish, this meant that the hospital of choice was Cedars-Sinai. There's a reason it's called the Hospital of the Stars, although truth be told I have never seen any famous people in all the times I've been there. It really is a beautiful complex though, with museum-quality art on every floor and every single kind of high-tech medical equipment imaginable. I saw quite a bit of all of it during my two pregnancies.

I didn't expect I'd have a high-tech birthing experience, although at the time I was kinda proud of it—to a point. Even though I opted for a hospital birth, my kid's birth was going to be natural, all the way. No drugs for me. Just me taking big cleansing breaths while having my husband there to cheer me on.

The first six months of my first pregnancy were fairly uneventful—no morning sickness to speak of and nothing unusual to report from my prenatal checkups. But around that six month mark a gigantic endocrinologic bomb exploded inside me. I gained weight—lots of it—and my normally petite face grew to the size of a pumpkin. My blood pressure was higher than it was supposed to be and I was this close to having gestational diabetes. If that wasn't bad enough, I also broke out with the worst case of acne and started growing a beard! My husband was pretty understanding about it, but I imagined this little baby-to-be was going to wish she could retreat back into that uterus when she got a look at this horrid, hairy, zit-filled face of her mother's.

Because of these changes in me, alarm bells rang out in my doctor's office and I was marched over to Cedars for twice-weekly stress tests. If you've never had one of these, don't worry; it's a simple test to make sure the baby's heart is beating normally, although telling the mother-to-be that it's a called a stress test doesn't do anything to calm the worried mind. Anyway, the good news was that while my outside was a mess, all this monitoring showed that everything inside was progressing nicely.

About a week before my due date, I was having one of these stress tests done when the nurse picked up the graph spewing from the printer and held it up to me with a big smile on her face. "Look, you're having contractions," she said, pointing to the sharp spiky black lines on the paper. I smiled too. I didn't feel a thing, and if this was what having contractions was all about, I was home free.

It was decided then—note that I had no say in this decision—that because of my precarious state and those contractions, I was to be induced. No rushing to get to the hospital, no packing bags, no having my water break naturally. No, I was calmly walked down the hall to the birthing area, and before I knew it I was on my back getting shot up with Pitocin and having my labor forced upon me.

As Betsy indicates, there is something about childbirth that makes a woman forget the pain involved. Yet on this first go-round, I had to conclude it wasn't all that bad. My Lamaze training paid off; all that breathing really *did* mask the pain of the contractions. Nine-and-a-half hours later, I was the proud mother of a healthy baby girl.

I also have to admit that I recovered from this birth rather quickly. Whether that was due to having been in good shape, good genes or those crazy hormones doing me a favor, I don't know. In any event, I went home the next day and shocked my very traditional mother when I drove to the supermarket the day after that. I felt fine and even went back to my low-impact aerobics class (hey, this is what everyone was doing then) three weeks later.

I'm not going to tell you that this is how it'll be for you. Every woman is different. All I can say is to listen to your body. She'll let you know when you're ready to return to your pre-pregnancy activities.

In my case, after a couple of months, the acne and the facial hair went away—as did the weight—and a few years later I was ready to do it again. Of course the second time around was totally different. This time the entire pregnancy was uneventful. My son was growing so well inside me that there was some concern he was growing *too* well. My doctor was concerned that his head was going to be the size of a small watermelon, too big to travel safely through the birth canal, meaning I would be forced to have a C-section. He consulted with a number of his Ivy League OB-GYN buddies, who came up with all kinds of ways to calculate the circumference of the baby's head and compare that to the width of my birth canal. They all reached the same conclusion. This baby had to come out sooner rather than later. I had an amniocentesis, which indicated he was ready to go. So there I was, marching back to the hospital two weeks before the due date, all so I could avoid a C-section. Once again I didn't get to experience having my water break. Once again I was induced, but not too worried. After all, the last go-round wasn't too bad.

Be careful what you wish for. This was *nothing* like the first time. About an hour into the induction, I had the worst case of back labor imaginable. Let me tell you. I hope none of you ever have to experience back labor. Being hit over the head with a sledgehammer would have felt better! No amount of Lamaze breathing was going to work this time. Just like that, my dreams of another natural birth went down the tubes. I wanted drugs—all of them. I begged for an epidural; the moment I felt that numbness over my lower body I felt ecstatic.

That feeling didn't last long, though. After hours of contractions and continuous measurement of my cervix, it became clear that this labor was going nowhere. Despite all those calculations, all that pre-planning and all those tests, I ended up having a C-section anyway. And that giant head my son was supposed to have? Well, that head turned out to be just as normal as the rest of him, although I do have to admit I was pretty surprised when he came out with blonde hair and blue eyes since both my husband and I are brunettes. Still, in the end I truly had nothing to complain about. I had a healthy newborn son.

That final thought is so important I feel like I need to repeat it. Whatever happens during your pregnancy, and whether you have a hospital birth, a home birth, whether you use a doctor or a midwife or a witch doctor, *none of that matters.* The only thing that counts is that tiny little bundle of love that you get to hold in your arms afterward. But having a good story to wrap around it makes it interesting.

Chapter 2
Bringing Home Baby

Betsy: Okay, so a baby literally just came out of your vagina (or in my case was cut out of my stomach). Either way you're sore and probably exhausted, but you rally for the big reveal.

I think it's funny that when you give birth in a hospital they are required to wheel you out in a wheelchair, but after that you're on your own. Some pre-birth advice I was given and thankfully heeded was to skip the homecoming party. Tell the relatives to wait a week, and go home and settle in with your baby. Remember all those plans you made for how labor was going to happen, which probably didn't pan out? Well, the homecoming is the same.

I know you dreamed of changing your baby into that beautiful new baby jumper, placing him or her into that brand new crib, and blissfully watching your little bundle of joy sleep—but the truth is, coming home is an adjustment. First of all, half the baby stuff you received still isn't assembled, or if it is, these days you'll need to read the instruction manual a few times to get it to work just right.

By Betsy Chasse and Debbie Spector Weisman

While maybe you've changed a few diapers already, this is *your* baby, not a niece or a nephew, and somehow it's different. In hindsight I've come to realize that these first few days of just you and your baby are going to tell you a lot about the road ahead.

Each of my children were different from the get-go. My daughter was on fire from the minute she was born, and she had no issues with communicating her needs and wants. Sleep? Well, yeah, that didn't happen. She was strong-willed from day one and is still going strong 11 years later. My son was chilled for the most part, but when he had a moment, he *had* one: a full-on, no holds barred, "one," and to this day that is exactly how he is. This really surprised me with all the talk about environment versus genetics, and of course there is a lot of truth to that. But I'll tell you what: that time with each of them, just us, helped me figure out a few things about who these babies were that came in handy later.

You learn to understand their cries, their sounds, their faces…and they learn too. After a few days of being cooped up in the house and recuperating from a C-section I wanted to take my baby for a walk—in that new, awesome stroller by the way. So we

It Came Out of my Vagina! Now What?!

packed up the stroller and the diaper bag and pretty much everything we could fit into the car and headed out to a local walking trail. Baby Elora was all smiles for the car ride and she even transferred to the stroller without a hitch. *Whoa this baby thing is gonna be easy,* I thought! For the first four minutes it was. Then we get about five minutes into our "look at our gorgeous family" walk, and my sweetly sleeping baby loses it. Out of nowhere she begins to cry like there is no tomorrow. I was in a panic. I didn't know this cry! I tried shifting the sun visor on the stroller. I tried giving her a binky…nope, nada. I finally take her out of the stroller and in an instant she is calm and back to sleep…hmmm, okay. So I give her a minute, then lay her back down in the stroller. Her head barely touched the cute little baby pillow and, "WAAAAAAA!" So I pick her up: "Ahhh," put her down, 'WAAAA." We did this for a few minutes when I realized it. This baby did not like my awesome, super chic, ridiculously overpriced, all-the-hip-moms-have-them stroller. Elora was not a stroller baby; Elora was a carry me or wear me baby. So much for my parading down Main Street strolling my baby.

By Betsy Chasse and Debbie Spector Weisman

By the time Elora was three, I had every type of baby-wearing contraption you could imagine. Eventually she got used to the stroller thing, but my learning on that sunny afternoon was: Honor your baby. Listen to your baby. Your baby is going to tell you exactly what she needs and wants, and taking the time early on to get to know her will make all the difference in the world as she grows.

If you're lucky, you received tons of gifts from your friends and relatives, along with all that unsolicited advice. Now comes the hard part. What do you do with all this stuff?

Essential Devices: For starters, there are the essentials, the things that you're most likely to actually use. Debbie and I agree on some, but not all, ultimately remember this, baby products are an industry and often times companies want to sell you stuff, stuff you probably don't need, keep it simple, the less you buy the lighter your diaper bag will be.

It Came Out of my Vagina! Now What?!

1. **Debbie: A good federally-approved crib:** this is the one that has rigid slats, not like the adjustable side crib I had with my kids. This is one of the good things about living today. Things that were unsafe and that we didn't know were unsafe are now banned from use. The generation before me—that means the crib I had when I was a baby—had slats that were so far apart a kid could put her head through it. So give yourself a pat on the back for being a mother today.

   Betsy: I co-slept with both my kids (OMG!) but I did have a crib, for nap time and when, well you know, the hubby and I wanted a little "alone" time. I did buy one of those little cribs that connected to the bed. It was great when they are newborn's and you're worried about rolling over and crushing them, but eventually they figured out how to wiggle their way right into the bed.

2. **Debbie: A good federally-approved car seat:** this is another device that has improved dramatically over the years. Today's seats easily move from car to carriage or stroller, which is a big

improvement over the past, when you had to pry your baby out of the seat and all those safety straps just so you could strap her into a stroller to get her into the house. This may not sound like much, but believe me, this is a godsend when you realize that not having to remove your child means not having to wake him up just to move from one place to another.

Betsy: Couldn't agree more with this one, it's a must have.

3. **Debbie: A stroller:** this is another example of technology on the move. They still make the cheap strollers that fold up like giant umbrellas, and they will do the job in a pinch. But you don't want that. You want the best stroller money can buy. Uh…on second thought, I take that back. Strollers are a lot like cars. You can get a stroller that costs nearly as much as a Maserati, but unless you're the type of person who has so much money she doesn't know what to do with it, a super fancy stroller is a super waste of money. Sure it's pretty, but you can get an awful lot of bells and whistles and a transport device that you'll be proud to push for hundreds of dollars less. Hopefully

one of your nice relatives already bought one of these for you. If not, shop around. There are tons of great choices out there. **Betsy**: Seriously, you can go broke buying a stroller and when all is said and done, it's the wheels that matter, are you active, do you like to run, go on long walks, or are you a mall walker, what's the weather like where you live, it's all about the wheels, consider your lifestyle and buy accordingly.

4. **Debbie: Baby bottles:** yes, I know. You're going to breastfeed. But you're going to need bottles for all those times you're too tired, or on one of those post-baby date nights you're required to keep your marriage alive (see Chapter 15). I'm not going to give you specific advice on which type of bottle to buy, since this is mostly a personal preference issue. Just realize that bottles literally come in all shapes, sizes, materials, and even different nipple designs. There are so many out there, there are almost too many to choose from. Some claim to reduce gas or prevent colic. Some maintain they're best for breast feeders, and some specifically market to

formula-fed babies. Some claim they're leak-free, easy to assemble, easy to clean. Yes, it's enough to make your head spin. Just make sure you buy a quality brand that's BPA-free. BPA is a type of plastic that we now know oozes carcinogens into the milk. Fortunately, all the bottle makers know this and because it's such a great marketing hook for nervous mothers like you, they're well-advertised and readily available.

Betsy: And along with this you'll want a bottle warmer, these things are handy. I tried the old school warm on the stove method, but it was time consuming and I was never sure if it was the right temperature. These things run about $20 bucks and are worth it.

5. **Debbie: Baby food processor:** I didn't have these when my kids were babies, and I wish I had. I might not have relied so much on all those jarred foods. Today's processors are so easy to use; I'm going to give you a guilt trip if you don't get one since this is the best way to ensure your little bundle of joy gets the most nutritious meals possible. All you have to do is put

some fresh food into the bowl, press a button and *voila!* Instant puree at the proper consistency and temperature.

Betsy: I think any old food processor works, a blender or anything like it will do the trick.

6. **Debbie: Changing table:** it's nice to have a piece of furniture in your nursery that's dedicated to the one job you'll have to do over and over on a daily basis for the next couple of years. If you can afford it, a changing table is a great thing. Chances are, though, that you're cramped for space or just don't have the luxury of that specific type of furniture. Fortunately, you don't need it. Today there are many makers of nice soft pads and pillows that sit on any flat surface and serve as a resting place for your baby while you clean up the waste created by that wonderful meal you made in that baby food processor (see above). Look for ones that are easy to clean or that come with removable washable covers.

Betsy: Yep, waste of money if you ask me, it looks nice and all, but a towel and a floor and a nice little basket which carries all your changing stuff works great. I preferred this with baby #2. I found a basket with 4 compartments, diapers, butt cream, wipes, cleaner and nail clipper. I kept 2, one upstairs and one down, saved about $500 bucks too.

7. **Debbie: Diapers:** I'm going to get in trouble on this one. I'm a big fan of disposable diapers. Their convenience to me outweighs their negative environmental impact. But let's face it. Getting rid of waste is an issue, any way you look at it. I have friends who swear by cloth diapers, and they believe they're doing the best thing for the environment by not adding all those tons of plastic to our already overflowing landfills. That may be true and I applaud their commitment and efforts. Then I think about all the carbon that gets spewed in the air from the electricity they're using to wash those diapers and I feel better.

Call me a Neanderthal. I recycle religiously, buy organic, and stay away from needless chemicals and additives. This is the one area where simple convenience trumps do-goodism. I don't want to have to wash loads of icky smelling diapers or pay a ton of money for a diaper service. I don't want to have to deal with the inevitable leaks that come with improper folding of cloth diapers. I want to get in there, swap out the dirty for the fresh with as little effort as possible. You don't like it? Tough.

Betsy: There are some good organic brands and you could get a diaper company for cloth diapers – look this is up to you, and don't feel bad if you're judged, a babies gotta poop, so there.

8. **Debbie: Baby monitor:** This is a convenience I like. There are tons of models out there, from simple audio devices to souped-up electronic video displays that present your baby in full living color. They come in two basic varieties—analog and digital. Digital devices can be encrypted, which means they're private, so there's no risk of your neighbor getting wind of your baby's cries from an errant sound wave. Analog products work off your Wi-Fi directly from the monitor to the receiver. Either kind might be subject to interference, but most of the time the

monitor does a great job of letting you know little Clarice is sleeping peacefully or that baby Jeremy is crying and in need of a diaper change.

Betsy: Okay, watch out because these things are addicting, I recall having a TV version and one night I put my baby to sleep and was looking forward to a quiet evening of TV and peace and then all I did was constantly stare at the monitor waiting for her to wake up, sometimes you need to turn it off and or move away from the device.

9. **Debbie: Baby carriers:** there are times when using a stroller is cumbersome, like when walking in a park or a crowd, and that's why baby carriers were invented. Again, lots of products out there, so personal preference is the deciding factor.

Betsy: I have to say I found this side sling, cheap too, like $14 at Target, it was the best one. The front carriers can wreak havoc on your back and the wraps, well okay I could not figure those things out, and I just kept worrying that my baby was going to fall out! I was never good at knots. Remember your baby is going to grow, so don't go broke buying these things as you're going to end up buying a few.

Non-essential devices: Companies that make products know they have a captive market with new mothers. You're so anxious to do the right thing, and so stressed out with all you have to do that you'll jump at the chance to purchase a product that purports to make your life easier. Because they know that and are out to make a buck for themselves, there's a cottage industry of devices that they want you to think are "must-haves" but, really, are things you can—and in some cases should—live without.

1. **Baby gyms**: A play pad is a great idea for a baby. But some people go overboard with elaborate contraptions that really don't do much to promote good athletic bones. There are even companies that want you to believe your kid needs dumbbells and exercise equipment. Some toys and attention are all you need at this stage.

By Betsy Chasse and Debbie Spector Weisman

2. **Crying analyzer:** These things tell you why your baby is crying. You'll figure this out fast enough without having to pay big bucks for it.

3. **Poop alarm:** Bells go off when the diaper is full. Believe me, it won't take long for you to figure this out without an added device.

4. **Baby perfume and baby heels:** I know kids grow up fast these days, but do we really have to start them out as adults while they're still infants?

5. **Car monitor:** This lets out an alarm when you leave your baby in the car. If you really need this product, you've got more problems than an errant child.

6. **Baby wigs:** Some kids are born with a head full of hair. Someone came up with the idea of doing something for those

who are follicly challenged. Only for those who can't tell when a grown man is wearing a toupee.

7. **Baby fan:** These aren't meant to cool off your baby on a hot, sunny day. Their intent is to dry off a wet bottom. Unnecessary.

8. **Baby mop:** Literally a mop attached to baby clothes. I thought child labor was banned over a century ago.

9. **Organic products:** I don't mean organic as in natural food or clothing. I mean things made from baby parts, like sculptures made from placentas and umbilical cords, and jewelry made from baby milk and baby hair. Yuck.

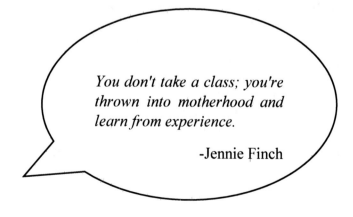

You don't take a class; you're thrown into motherhood and learn from experience.

-Jennie Finch

By Betsy Chasse and Debbie Spector Weisman

Chapter 3
Surviving Other Family Members

> "And....while she did help clean the house 'a bit' (I am super particular and we had a bitch of a shaggy wool rug...) after my son was born, she helped focus on my needy dog - walked, fed and slept with him at night- so he too could adjust to the new bundle of joy that entered "his" house."
>
> ~ Erica, Debbie's grown-up daughter

Betsy: Remember how in Chapter 2, I said you should keep your relatives away for at least a week? Well you're going to need that time for sure, because once that week is over it's hello Mom, Mothers-in-law, Aunties, Uncles, Sisters-in-law and best friends (who've already had babies mostly—let's face it, you're probably going to lose most of your babyless friends anyway, so get used to it). All of them will want to check out the newest member of your family, and while most won't admit it, they will check out your mommy skills as well.

You've heard the horror stories and for the most part, sadly, they are true. Once the in-laws get ahold of that baby, the only time they are going to give him back is when his diaper stinks or he's crying, and then they are going to tell you how to fix it. This isn't some old cliché, it's fact. It's as if these normally loving and wonderful women all of a sudden become possessed know-it-alls, unable to keep their pie holes shut.

I can say this because I have been there, and to be fair, have been one myself. (Hell, I'm writing this book aren't I!) The truth is, everyone means well; they just want you to be happy and your baby to be happy, and they hope sharing their horror stories will save you the frustrations, angst and whatever else they went through.

There are a few ways you can deal with this phenomenon, and some work better than others. I highly suggest you skip throwing that bottle of freshly pumped breast milk in their faces, because let's be real—that's what we'd all like to do, right?

By Betsy Chasse and Debbie Spector Weisman

1. Limit the time! This is actually the easiest thing to do. If your family wants to visit from out of town – limit it to one or two weeks, maximum. Having a time limit helps you to know that there is a light at the end of that tunnel and most of us can manage two weeks even under these hard circumstances.

2. If you're using one or more of your family members for child care, set the ground rules and stick to them. If you want your baby to sleep in the yellow jammie set then by god he/she will or they are out. Remember this is your baby and if they ignore your simple rules, then they are probably ignoring the important ones. In the end paying for child care may feel expensive, but your head and your heart and your peace of mind will be better off for it. This is going to be the hardest part, and for me I suggest avoiding it unless it's absolutely necessary. I don't mean Grandma and that Great Aunt can't take Junior out for a day or two, but counting on them full time can put an unneeded burden on the relationship. And when they do take them out—well, guess what? Unless they are belly up

to the local bar with your baby in tow, let them do it the way they want! You survived, didn't you? Just like you want to parent the way you feel most comfortable, they should have the same respect. So if you're going to go full out with the in-law day care, then you're going to have to be reasonable and get clarity *before* the baby is born.

3. Don't be afraid to sit the usually loving offender down and communicate about the issue. I know, who wants to talk about it? But honest and open communication often clears up any misunderstandings early on and saves everyone the trouble of hearing about it later from your other sister. (Gossip can make for very ugly family gatherings and festering resentment smells worse than a day old cloth diaper). If you don't have this kind of relationship with that in-law caring for your kid…then again, they shouldn't be doing it.

4. Grin and bear it. For those short visits where in the light of all eternity just smiling like a Cheshire cat and nodding will make the afternoon easier on everyone, do that. In the end, who gives

a poop what they say? You only have to let it make you feel "less than" if you want to. Otherwise, in one ear and out the other!

I've said it before; the truth is, if they are in your life and you are letting them around you and your baby, even the most annoying of mothers-in-law means well. You know who you're dealing with so act accordingly. Set the ground rules early. It's likely you and your significant other have already dealt with the pushiest of in-laws, so have a refresher conversation with your spouse about your boundaries and don't bother cleaning the house.

As a matter of fact, my last piece of advice is: let them come, let them cook and let them clean. All you have to do is sit in that new baby rocker with your boppy and your baby and be served.

It Came Out of my Vagina! Now What?!

> *"Having a baby changes the way you view your in-laws. I love it when they come to visit now. They can hold the baby and I can go out."*
>
> -Matthew Broderick quotes

Debbie: Okay, it's my time to chime in here. There is one very, very important exception to this, and this is a very, very special case: the mom who's really good at helping out.

I can speak to this from both ends. I don't know how I would have managed those first weeks of motherhood without my mom helping out, and I know I was very much appreciated being that kind of grandma to my newborn grandson.

I knew from my two older sisters' experiences that having my mother around when I got home from the hospital would be a good thing. We all had had contentious relationships with her, for varying reasons, but when it came to caring for her grandchildren she really knew how to shine. This was ironic, since she had a nurse when all three of us were babies, so I don't know where she picked up all the newborn mothering skills. *But she had them.* She taught me how to properly put on a diaper, how to give an infant a bath, how warm to heat the bottles, and all that stuff you're supposed to know but don't.

My mom flew in from her home in Florida and we were fortunate enough to have a spare room for her. I think she stayed for about six or seven weeks. She did everything. She cooked, she cleaned (oh boy did she clean; I couldn't leave a bread crumb without her standing behind me with a paper towel to scoop it up.) In later visits when the kids were older I would find the cleaning part to be a bit overbearing. No, scratch that, a lot overbearing. But in those early days of motherhood, I was grateful for all the help I could get.

My mother was also a great knitter, and while she wasn't tending to the baby, she was busily making sweaters and baby blankets. If you've ever checked out the cost of hand-knit baby stuff, you know the great bargain I got here. Mind you, I wasn't exaggerating about the great knitter part. We're talking heirloom quality here, and I was very grateful to get it.

It was also great to have her around when my son was born, as she made a great babysitter for my daughter while we were at the hospital. Again, she stayed several weeks to see me through those early days. This was especially helpful when it came to my son's *bris*.

For those who may not know, a bris is the Jewish ritual of circumcision that happens when the boy is eight days old. While neither my husband nor I were very religious, we never once considered not doing this for our son. It was also something that was done at the house, and since it was a Jewish event that, of course, meant lots and lots of people and lots and lots of food.

Although my mother was a pretty good cook, we weren't going to force her to prepare food for this event, so we hired a caterer. She took care of overseeing this, as she refused to let me get out of bed and overexert myself. I had a C-section with my son, and she wanted me to get as much rest as possible.

By Betsy Chasse and Debbie Spector Weisman

I, on the other hand, felt perfectly fine. On the day of the bris, I got up, took a shower, put on makeup and my best-fitting dress. After all, we were having a party and I wanted to look my best.

My mother looked at me like I was nuts. "Why are you doing out of bed?" she asked. "You have to take care of yourself."

"I am taking care of myself," I grumbled. "I'm getting ready for our guests."

She was even more horrified when I walked into the living room to witness the event. "You shouldn't be watching this," she warned. I suppose I should have been mortified by the thought of having my son's foreskin ripped apart, but I wasn't.

I looked up and noticed that every woman in the room over 40 was giving me that same evil-eye look. *What are you doing up? You ought to be in bed.*

Personally, that conjured up an image in my head of a Nineteenth Century invalid wallowing under her bedsheets, whispering, "Oh woe is me," over and over. I was a modern woman and having none of that. If there was going to be a party in my house, I was all in. That is, as long as I could act like a guest and not have to do any work. I had just given birth, after all.

I won out and got to see my son get circumcised. I took it a lot better than my husband, who nearly fainted when the *mohel* did the deed. We were fortunate that his father was holding the baby at the time. Oh yes, that reminds me. We hosted both my mother and my father-in-law that week. Fortunately, that was such a long time ago that the memory of how stressful that combination was has long since passed.

On the flip side, I flew in to be with my daughter when my grandson was born. She had scheduled things so that her mother-in-law was to be there for the birth and I would come to help her afterward. Of course, it didn't quite work out that way. That little boy waited days after his due date to be born, and since I had booked my flight in advance, I got there before the birth and she had to play hostess to both her mother and her mother-in-law. Fortunately, she chose to work right up till the day before she went to the hospital, so she was able to manage having both of us at the same time. Also, I have to admit, for two mothers-in-law and about-to-be-grandmothers, we behaved almost like reasonably mature adults.

She, too, ended up with an unplanned C-section, and I think she appreciated having that extra help in those first days. My husband drove up while they were in the hospital and she was grateful to have him there. Her mother-in-law left soon after that, but I stayed around for three more weeks. This time *I* was the one doing the cooking and cleaning (though not much), and I was around to give her and my son-in-law a date night two weeks after the birth. A week later, my husband came back in time for all of us to celebrate the baby's first Thanksgiving.

Family can be a pain or they can be a blessing and sometimes they can be both. As long as everyone knows their role in advance, everyone wins.

Chapter 4
Feeding Facts and Myths

Debbie: When I was a new parent, I based my global philosophy on one simple truth: do the opposite of what my mom did. Now my mom was a very nice person and was a terrific grandmother, and this isn't really a slam against her. It was just that at the time I wasn't too happy about the way I turned out, so I thought there had to be a better way.

This was especially true when it came to food. I grew up as a very picky eater. My lunchbox staples were peanut butter sandwiches and jelly sandwiches. Mind you, I didn't say peanut butter and jelly. No, I hated them in combination, but as separate and equal participants they had a high rank in my daily caloric intake. (By the way, the shortcut PB&J is a modern invention. I never heard that term in my growing up years.) The only vegetables I ate were carrots and celery sticks and the occasional green beans that I only ate raw, never cooked. Fruits, too, were a no-no, their brands of sweetness for some reason a complete turn off for me.

No, my food source of choice was sugar. That's right, that element that we now know as an evil addictive demon of destruction was the most exalted item on my own personal food pyramid. At breakfast I ate every brand of sugar-coated cereal on the market, and when the cereal came without obvious sugar—say, Cheerios for example—I'd add a solid two teaspoons of sugar to the bowl before taking my first bite. On weekends, my father would treat us with waffles, which of course couldn't be consumed without a heaping portion of delicious artificial-flavored maple syrup.

This obsession with sweetness didn't end with the obvious sources. The only way my mom could get me to eat scrambled eggs was with syrup on top. Just the thought of that alone now adds inches to my waistline, but it's the truth. I really liked it that way.

During my school years, not a day went by that I didn't come home to a chocolate milkshake, again made with love by my mom. I'd usually use it to wash down my other late afternoon snack—

It Came Out of my Vagina! Now What?!

Melody cookies. These chocolate cookies—sprinkled on top with sugar—were a big seller among the Baby Boom generation and I'll never know why Nabisco decided to stop selling them. Was it because they were sugar on top of sugar? Perhaps. But I can remember eating boxes of them at a time.

The second biggest part of my diet was fat. If you take a look at my name it's pretty obvious I'm of the Hebrew persuasion. I grew up in a Kosher home, and that meant lots of traditional Jewish cooking. By definition, this ethnic food is infused with tons and tons of exquisitely delicious food that is made tasty by its super extra quota of fat. We didn't eat bacon but my mom made beef fry—slabs of fatty meat fried to tasty crispness. Mashed potatoes were flavored with fat, too. Not with butter, which is bad enough, but with chicken fat, a particularly artery-clogging version. In fact, one of my mom's delicacies—something she learned from *her* mother—was an appetizer known by its Yiddish name *gribenes*, which means fried chicken skins cooked in *schmaltz,* which is a fancy way of saying artery-clogging chicken fat. I ate this stuff by the bowlful, and somehow I'm still around to tell you about it.

By Betsy Chasse and Debbie Spector Weisman

Let's not even talk about all the trips to the deli for hot corned beef and hot pastrami sandwiches; the fatter the meat, the tastier the treat. How I didn't end up with diabetes or become a 400-pound blob of mush by the time I was ten is nothing short of a miracle.

I wasn't going to have my kids suffer this same fate. No siree, my kids were going to be prime examples of perfect nutrition from the get-go. Three squares of balanced meals, no artificial ingredients, and—drumroll please—no added sugar.

I don't remember how long this commitment lasted, but looking back at photos of my daughter's face covered with gooey chocolate cake icing at her first birthday party makes me believe it didn't last very long. Believe me, I know I tried. Back then if there was any commercially available organic baby food around, I didn't know about it. But I tried very hard to stay away from giving my kids too much processed food. I did a lot of cooking and always had a fresh bowl of fruit on the kitchen counter.

I still have the cookbooks I bought detailing how to make healthy baby food and nutritious snacks your kids will love. There are a few food-stained pages in them, but not many. Most of the recipes were untouched and untried.

Why did I give up? I was determined to cook healthy meals for my kids. I didn't want to be one of those moms whose idea of a meal plan was whatever frozen food was on sale this week at Ralph's. They would get beautiful hand-crafted meals made with good, natural ingredients and sprinkled with love on top.

There was only one problem—getting them to eat it.

The turning point came after one incident that will forever be imprinted on my cooking mind. That was the day I decided to treat them to something that by definition is not the most healthful of dishes, but at least would be made more so by eliminating the artificial ingredients and preservatives found in the commercial product: homemade macaroni and cheese. (This is another example of today's shortening of terms to their basics. Back then it was never called mac and cheese.) Anyway, I found a wonderful recipe in one of those back-to-nature cookbooks. I forget what brand of whole wheat macaroni I used or what kind of super fresh cheese made it into the casserole dish, but in the end it didn't matter. Even though it looked great and to my palate tasted delicious, I couldn't get either of my little darlings to swallow down more than that first bite which they both, surprisingly, spit back out on their plates.

Their simultaneous "Yuck!" brought tears to my eyes. How could I raise two young children to a healthy adulthood if they preferred Kraft to my well-intentioned plans?

It only got worse from there. Yes, I was one of those moms who made McDonald's a staple of our diet with one, maybe two—dare I say three—weekly trips to the Golden Arches. Sad to say, I have the proof too. When cleaning out their rooms of their childhood collectibles, I found enough Happy Meal toys to fill a giant banker's box. I justified it at the time by telling myself that the exercise they got from playing at the McDonald's indoor playground would burn off those wasteful calories. And let's face it, those fries were delicious. I'd be lying if I said I didn't swallow my own share of fast food fare.

But I got lucky. Neither of my children developed any dread diseases from eating any of this stuff. Nor did they turn into the humongous blob I thought I'd be from my all-sugar youth diet. Chalk it up to great metabolisms or great genes or that benevolent spirit in the sky that determined my kids would be spared any ill effects of bad diet. They made it to adulthood with healthy bodies and healthy minds.

You know what else they brought to their adulthood? The belief that they weren't going to live it with the diet their mother "imposed" on them. Uh-uh. My kids now crave healthy food. My daughter, who very early on just decided she didn't like meat, is not quite a vegetarian but buys all her food at Trader Joe's and Whole Foods. She makes all of my grandson's food, and as a result, that evil taste of sugar has never entered his lips. How long she can keep that up is anyone's guess, but all power to her for now. My son has become a connoisseur of kombucha and infused Chai teas, and except for the occasional pizza, eats a very healthy diet.

My moral here is simple: Do what I say, not what I do. Here's my program on how to feed your child in the 21st Century:

By Betsy Chasse and Debbie Spector Weisman

1. Don't introduce sugar into your child's diet.
2. Read labels. Don't buy anything at the supermarket that has words on the label you can't pronounce.
3. Buy only organic and fresh vegetables and fruit.
4. Don't feed your child any red meat. But if you must, do so sparingly.
5. Make water the drink of choice. Ban all sodas and processed juices from your life.
6. Do not eat any GMO foods. And if you don't know what a GMO food is, you shouldn't be reading this book.
7. Ban all white flour from their diet.
8. Pizza is a four letter word. (Okay, it's got five letters, but who's counting.)
9. Get a juicer and make your own vegetable juices.
10. If you must indulge in sweets, buy a cookbook that shows you how to make brownies out of beans and cookies out of rice flour.
11. Finally, and this is the most important one of all: *don't feel like a failure if you can't maintain this regimen*. Society is against

you. Television is against you. The Internet is against you. Your kids' peers are against you. Good for you if you try, but remember one thing: that Oreo won't kill your kid.

> *"I want my children to have all the things I couldn't afford. Then I want to move in with them."*
>
> -Phyllis Diller

Betsy: Before I get into the actual food (as in solid foods) part of feeding time, let's talk a little bit about the other type of food your baby is going to consume in the early stages of their life...the liquid kind. The one that for the most part comes out of your boobs, and for many, gets mixed up in a bottle.

First off, the reality is—if you're going to breast feed, then tell your partner the boobs are off-limits. Okay yes, there are a kinky few who like to partake in the baby's elixir, but to me that's just gross. So sorry if I'm judgmental. It honestly gives me the weebie jeebies just thinking about it.

Anyway, I digress. The first thing you need to decide is: am I going to breast feed or bottle feed? Sometimes this choice is up to you and sometimes it's not.

For the record I highly recommend breastfeeding, if you can. Yes, you're finally going to have cleavage bigger than a Playmate; yes, at one point you're going to leak milk all over your favorite shirt while out to dinner with the gang and your best girlfriend is going to give you that weird eye maneuver (you know, from your eyes to your breasts) until you realize you just leaked Johnny's dinner onto your foie gras; and yep, your boobs will no longer be yours until you decide you've had enough. You will become an expert in bathroom pumping and feeding (I got really good at walking and feeding).

I was lucky. Breastfeeding came easy to me and my babies, but that is not always the case. I highly suggest meeting with a lactation consultant, and am about to contradict myself here. Usually I'm telling you to tell people to butt out, but the truth is, asking for help from the right people could make all the difference, and this is one of those instances. There are some nifty tricks (ancient secrets, actually) that when passed along can save you a lot of frustration and keep you from upsetting your boobs. Seriously—getting it right will save your boobs from a lot of pain, and your heart too.

But if, after a good try, you aren't able to breastfeed, well, guess what? That is totally awesome, too. I'd like to take this moment to remind you that you created life—yeah, *life*—you know, the most amazing process in the world. You just did that, so whether you breastfeed your baby or feed them from a Yak's bladder, seriously it's not worth the upset. This does not in any way diminish your amazing value as a mother.

If you decide to use formula for any other reason, the same applies. You created life, so everyone can take their judgment and shove it. Period.

However, if you breastfeed, you do have to watch your diet. Pretty much everything you eat, your baby eats. If your baby is fussy then start with your diet. Go back to that lactation consultant or a nutritionist, and begin to eliminate foods until you figure out what's bugging your baby's tummy. Babies' tummies can be sensitive.

After I gave birth to my daughter, I was starving. Remember that giant labor I went through? That meant I had not eaten in almost two days! All I wanted was a big plate of veggies, thinking this would be a great first meal for my baby. I piled up on all the cruciferous veggies I could find. At the time, a vegetable was a vegetable to me, and that meant it was healthy and nutritious. Only one little problem with that: I didn't realize cruciferous veggies also had a tendency to make one gassy. When I arrived for my first night home with baby she wailed for about four hours straight. It took a week or so to figure out that her tummy didn't like gassy veggies. Be patient (I know—with a screaming baby that's nearly impossible, but don't give up).

If you go for formula, then choose one that's organic. You could even join a breast milk co-op (yes they have those) and buy breast milk from some awesome woman who's sharing hers. There are a million options available to you. And I hate to tell you, but this is just one of the many millions of decisions you're going to make over your child's life. Do some research, make a choice and move on. I promise your baby is going to survive and it's unlikely that when they are in therapy later in life, it's going to come out that the reason for all their suffering is because you either didn't breastfeed, or you did. Nope they'll have much better ammunition by then.

Okay, now on to the solid food. I have a confession to make. I was one of those moms who puréed her own baby food picked directly from my garden. Yep, annoying, I know, but the truth is, I had that kind of lifestyle. Not everyone does, so again, stop beating yourself up over it. Buy the best baby food you can, preferably organic.

I fed both my babies exactly the same way—no sugar, an all organic, veggie-based diet, slowly introducing healthy organic foods—and guess what? My daughter has an amazing palate, will try just about anything, and yep, she loves a good cupcake. My son eats nothing but beige food, thinks veggies will kill him (I'm not exaggerating) and again, loves a good cupcake.

By Betsy Chasse and Debbie Spector Weisman

Food for kids isn't so much about taste as it is about texture. You can go ahead and make that veggie smiley plate, but your kids are going to eat what they like and that's it. Trying to force feed them healthy veggies is only going to give them a food complex. The best thing you can do is make healthy food available at every meal and snack and allow them to choose. Empowering your child to make healthy choices will be better for them in the long run. I have found there are a lot of healthy beige foods by the way, and I am not worried about my son's health at all. He's like an ox, that kid! I have heard it said and am here to agree: it's amazing how our kids survive on how little they actually eat, but they do. Teaching them to know when they are hungry and not bored, when they are full and how to find out what they like is more important than whether or not they eat their veggies at every meal. They will figure it out.

The other thing that eventually happens to our kids is they leave the house. (Yep, it's true. You can't keep them locked up inside till they're old enough to drive.) They observe what other kids are eating. This is a good thing and a bad thing. It's great when they see their best buddy eating carrots and decide they like them too (this happened to my son with carrots.) But it's a tough thing when they go to a party and the only drink available is soda, which is a no-no in our house. I've decided balance is best here. My kids know that soda is off-limits, but when we're at Jo Jo's birthday party and that's all they've got, well it *is* a party. Same goes for cake and candy.

Here's the thing I've learned: the more you say no, the more they want it, they crave it, and they pursue it (this pretty much works for about everything by the way). But educating them on why it's not good for them and why you're saying no goes a long way too. For the most part (save for a few *Mommy I just want it because I want it* meltdowns) reasoning with kids starting at around age four actually works. Before that they don't really know what they're missing.

By Betsy Chasse and Debbie Spector Weisman

Chapter 5
What?! You Didn't Pre-register for Daycare the Moment You Got Pregnant?

Debbie: What made me pick the preschool where I sent my daughter? A pony named Shadow.

Yep, after all the books I'd read, the literature handed out to me, and all the mailers that were sent by schools who somehow knew I had a toddler in the house (this was way before the Age of the Internet, by the way), I let a horse decide my child's educational future.

How did it come to this? Well, we have to start at the beginning...

Here's a little fun fact that nobody knows about me: I'm a professional parent. It's true. I have a document that says so and everything.

It Came Out of my Vagina! Now What?!

Shortly after my daughter was born I got caught up in the "creating your genius" baby movement. I found out about a course that was being given about fifty miles from my house that purported to guarantee that I could teach my baby to read and do math before she was out of diapers. What new mother could resist this?

I don't remember exactly how long the course lasted, but I do remember several trips up and down the freeway and getting drilled by people who were 1000% convinced their way was the *only* way. If everyone in America carried out their program, we'd have a country of super overachieving children who'd do everything from finding a cure for cancer to making the NBA all-star team at 16.

As a new, naïve mother desperate to do the right thing, I ate it all up. I went home and made myself dozens of flash cards, with everything on them from musical instruments to famous art paintings, to countries and, of course, the Presidents of the United States. At least three times a day, I'd sit my daughter in her infant seat—she was too young to sit up by herself—and run words and pictures past her blank, expressionless face. She had to be absorbing all this. They told me she was taking it in. I'd know for sure when she started talking.

I kept this up for quite some time. I even bought the flash cards they made for math, with dots representing the numbers up to 100. Each day I'd go through the routine, flashing cards past her face as fast as I could. They said she'd only need a nanosecond for each image to be imprinted on her memory, and by the time she was four she'd be doing calculus. I so was pleased I was giving her this vast data bank, and had visions of the next Marie Curie sleeping so peacefully in that crib.

Then one day I stopped. Was I getting bored with the process? Perhaps. It got tiring constantly whizzing those cards back and forth with no real feedback. I was also doing this in a vacuum, as none of my friends were sold on the idea. I began to wonder if I was doing it right—whether flashing ten cards at a time was too little or twenty too many. Was I showing her the right images to stimulate her brain cells? Could I get the same effect just by reading her books I was reading to her anyway?

It Came Out of my Vagina! Now What?!

Or maybe it was as simple as this: when she started to crawl she wouldn't sit still for these sessions. Well, that's not exactly true. Sometimes she did. But often she didn't, and that inconsistency helped dampen my enthusiasm for the process.

Whatever the reason, it doesn't matter. The moment I stopped I forever stripped her of her ability to rise to the top. I stomped out her potential to be the next Eleanor Roosevelt or Frida Kahlo or Emily Dickinson. I put a smear on the title of professional parent.

Or did I? I'm not going to go into the pros and cons of teaching methods or whether I really screwed up my daughter's life. (I fear I must inject a note of seriousness here. In truth, she's grown up to be extremely successful in business as well as a terrific mother and wife.) In the end, I did what every good parent strives to do—my best. I gave her my attention and my love. I filled the house with all sorts of "educational" toys and books and, in effect, spun the wheel and hoped it came up with success.

When it came time for preschool I did my due diligence. I got a list of all the recommended preschools in the area and went to visit them. The Montessori school seemed nice and it was very

By Betsy Chasse and Debbie Spector Weisman

close to my house, but something about it just didn't click. Another highly touted school turned me off when I saw them feeding the kids snacks of what looked to me like very rotten bananas.

A lot of my Jewish friends were opting for the preschools run by the area temples and synagogues. They all had excellent reputations, but I rejected them out of hand because I was still in my "I'm resisting religion" stage. At a very young age I'd been indoctrinated in Jewish law by a bunch of zealots whom I felt perverted the spirit of the religion. I wasn't going to do the same thing to my kids.

In the end, it came down to the preschool that offered pony rides on their campus. All the other preschools seemed to be offering the same mix of reading, art projects, playground equipment and such, but I liked the idea of my kid being able to ride on a pony every day. I mean, how cool is that!

Actually, it ended up being a very cool idea. She loved the pony, Shadow, naturally enough. Even more importantly, she loved the school. In addition to the animals, they provided a very solid early childhood education program that had her reading at three. She made lots of friends, one of whom she is still friends with to this day. I later found out that one of her classmates was the niece of a world leader, who actually paid several visits to the school in the time she was there.

Later on in this chapter, Betsy will relate her travels through the public school system of a major metropolitan city. I opted not to take that route. I'd heard lots of stories about how terrible the public schools were at the time, and I certainly didn't want to subject my daughter to all that. I had the means to pay for private school and since we were all so happy with the pony place, it was a no-brainer to let her stay there for kindergarten and elementary school.

I felt validated in that decision when I picked her up from school. Each time she'd get into the car I'd ask that question, "What did you do in school today?" Every day she'd always smile and reply, "I played." Given the homework she got every night, I knew it was more involved than that, but I was glad she loved the educational practice.

By Betsy Chasse and Debbie Spector Weisman

Things weren't quite so simple when it came to my son. This school wasn't a good fit for him from the get-go, and I had to switch him out to a more traditional preschool that had small classes and a teacher who could handle his super-energetic behavior. It was okay, since by the time he came around, old Shadow had been put out to pasture and the pony rides had stopped.

But by the time he came around, there was something new in our lives that really changed everything: computers. I know it's impossible to believe, but there was a time when computers didn't exist. My husband and I were actually kind of on the cutting edge, having bought our first computer several years before there was such a thing as Apple. Our pride and joy was a portable computer called the Osborne that looked like a small suitcase and had 64k of memory. That's right 64*k*, on two floppy disks, 32k for the program and 32k for the data with a teeny tiny 4-inch screen in the middle. It sounds crazy to think about now, but it really worked. I wrote twelve books on that machine, and it was a trusty little workhorse that served me well.

It Came Out of my Vagina! Now What?!

This was the computer that resided in our house when our daughter was born, but sadly, it wasn't made for baby or children's programs. That came a few years later when the Commodore 64 came out. Both my daughter and son gladly ate up the programs that a few enterprising computer nerds developed for that machine. I don't know how educational they really were, but the one program they loved the most was the one that taught them how to write their names by turning them into an animated movie that exploded all over the screen.

That truly was the dark ages as far as electronic gadgets go. Today I couldn't even begin to list all the ways you can use computers and tablets and smartphones to engage your little one. Today's babies are born with the knowledge that a smartphone is an extension of your hand and it's very likely that the first smile you get is not going to be aimed at you, but at your screen.

Yes, the world has changed greatly since my early parenting days, but some things do remain constant. Here are my top ten recommendations for creating the path to your own super baby's genius:

By Betsy Chasse and Debbie Spector Weisman

1. You will always be your baby's best teacher. Those big eyes looking up at you are constantly begging, "Teach me, Mommy."

2. Always talk to your baby. Even if you feel like a madwoman prattling around saying things like, "Here I am wiping down the kitchen counter with a towel," your baby is listening. I'm not a scientist and I don't have all the statistics, but it's been proven that the more you speak to your child before the age of one, the greater her/his capacity for language will be.

3. Read. Read. Read. If you do nothing else, getting your kids to love books is the best way to instill the love of education. Plus, you might learn a thing or two yourself.

4. The world is a school. Think of it. Your kid comes into life with a blank slate. Expose him/her to everything life has to offer. Let that brain fill up with the glories of this world. Stroll

through an art gallery; go to an outdoor concert, a sporting event, and the zoo. This is one area where you can't go wrong.

5. Get your kid into preschool. Unfortunately, there's no nationwide mandatory preschool education in this country, so you're gonna have to pay for it. Do your homework and seek out the best preschool you can afford.

6. Put limits on the electronics. Although I believe that FaceTime is the greatest gift in the world for grandparents, having your kid stare at a screen for hours on end will stunt his social and physical growth. Create a set schedule or set a timer on the computer, television, video game or smartphone. Insist on getting her butt outside to play and, if you have to, set up regular play dates. Chances are, those moms also have kids who'd rather play with their Pokemon pals than their real ones.

7. Trust your gut. If you're too confused by the choices in front of you, let your intuition be your best guide. It's usually right,

even if—like my experience with the pony school—it may seem illogical.

8. Unless you're hell-bent on getting your kid into Harvard, most choices in front of you will do your child well. Don't feel you've blown it if you can't get your kid into what others believe to be "the best." The right school for your kid may end up having a greater educational benefit than forcing him into the flavor-of-the-year school where he might end up feeling like a misfit.

9. Keep on top of things. Just because you drop your kid off at the door doesn't mean you're done. Keep close track of your child's progress. Have an open dialogue with the teacher, and don't feel intimidated. Speak up if you see problems developing.

10. In education as in real estate, it's all about location, location, location. Unless you're going private or homeschooling, make

school quality the most important criterion when choosing where to live. Once you get into elementary school, quality does matter, and this choice will have a major impact on your child's educational development.

11. (Okay, I said 10 but you're not really counting, are you?) Teach your children ethics. Kids don't automatically know the difference between right and wrong. They have to be shown it. Teach by example by living a life of integrity. Show them what it means to have empathy, sympathy, compassion. Whether you believe it or not, they are watching you constantly and because they love you they will want to emulate you in every way.

12. Really understand your child. It's natural to want your child to follow in your footsteps, but if she doesn't have the same love for Early Japanese Poetry as you do, don't see her as a failure. Pay attention to your child's strengths and seek out ways to

nurture them. Trying to mold them into a mini-you is likely to result in rebellion, mistrust and maybe worse.

> "The fastest way to break the cycle of perfectionism and become a fearless mother is to give up the idea of doing it perfectly - indeed to embrace uncertainty and imperfection."
>
> -Arianna Huffington

Betsy: I was lucky with my first child. I lived in the country and was involved in a group that had a preschool—cheap, fun and easy…whew! I had dodged the preschool bullet, until, that is, I moved from my little country estate to the big city. I made this move right as my son turned three, and upon our first visit to our new park a new mommy friend asked, "So what pre-school are you sending him to?"

"Ooh," I said. "I hadn't even thought of that, with moving from one state to another and all."

It Came Out of my Vagina! Now What?!

This mommy looked at me as if I had just cut out my child's heart and eaten it. "Oh, no," she said, "you're not even on a list?"

No, I wasn't on any lists; preschool wasn't even on my radar. Guilt and shame filled my body and I felt as though I'd just killed any chance of my son being the next leader of the free world. In big cities especially, most parents in the know register their kids for the "right" pre-school at conception. The moment that stick turns positive the mommies with the mostest are signing up for the right preschools, mommy and me classes, summer camps, and have on file the college application forms for their high achieving fetuses.

I was clearly behind schedule. I raced home and began the search. Thankfully the new mommy friend gave me a list of where my little guy should be going. I called them all and found out that not only was I last on the list, but most of these pre-schools cost more than one year of college (state college, but seriously!). I not only didn't have that kind of money, I couldn't fathom spending it on finger painting and sand box toys.

By Betsy Chasse and Debbie Spector Weisman

I sat in utter despair at what to do. In my search I had found a little tyke gymnastic class that everyone said was cool, so I signed him up for that, figuring at least he'll learn to roll over on his head or something. To my surprise, that kids' gym had just started a preschool. Better yet, they had space and I signed my guy up.

That decision turned out to be the best thing I'd ever done. My son loved the teacher, it was small (only four kids), and it started at 9am and went until 2pm! Most preschool programs are only in session for three hours daily (okay for the record $1200 a month for three hours a day is thievery!) That barely gives most moms time to drop the kid off, do a yoga class and go pick them up, leaving both parties tired and cranky and hungry.

What's the take away for me? Preschool is as much for mommy as it is for the kid. So find one that works for *both* of you! Make sure it has a diverse group of kids and that you can get along with the parents. These people are probably going to be in your life for a while; if you can't stand hanging out with them while your little ones play, then you're going to suffer. One can only pretend they haven't seen that episode of *Dora the Explorer* so many times

It Came Out of my Vagina! Now What?!

before it's clear you're avoiding "grown up" conversation. Kids are pretty easy to make happy, but if you're miserable, it won't be worth it.

Chapter 6: Managing Their Meltdowns...and Yours

> *"When my kids become wild and unruly, I use a nice, safe playpen. When they're finished, I climb out."*
>
> ~ Erma Bombeck

Betsy: By the time my daughter was 16-months-old, she had traveled more than most people will in their lifetime. We had the travel thing pretty much down pat. She could even manage a transatlantic flight with my boobs, a binky and her favorite pink blanket, lovingly referred to as *Sa Sa* (eventually Softy).

The only part of the travel experience that proved stressful was going through the security checkpoint, where everything (post 9-

It Came Out of my Vagina! Now What?!

11 everything) had to be X-rayed—including the binky and her precious *Sa Sa*. I tried many tricks to make this an easy three minutes of separation, but the reality was that she was no dummy. She anticipated this parting and decided she did not like it. Let's face it, who likes practically disrobing in the middle of an airport and shoving your beloved belongings onto a conveyer belt to who knows where? She may have anticipated the letting go, but I don't think she understood where it was going and if she would get it back, so traumatic it was, every time.

I tried to minimize the ear-piercing wailing by taking said *Sa Sa* and binky right at the very last minute and handing them to the TSA workers. The workers usually understood my weird hand gestures and wide eyes, but once in the Burbank Airport, a woman behind me wasn't so understanding. As we waited in line, I made my usual attempts at explaining to my little dear that in a few minutes we were going to give the man *Sa Sa* and binky but that we would get it back, I promise. As usual, the moment I pulled binky from her mouth, the cry was louder than a jet engine at take-off. As she screamed bloody murder I pried *Sa Sa* from her hands

By Betsy Chasse and Debbie Spector Weisman

and off it went into the abyss. I swear you'd think I just killed her kitten. I rushed through the X-ray machine myself and waited desperately on the other side for her treasures to reappear and amazingly enough, I heard through the cries of despair a woman behind me say "Oh My God can't you control your child?!"

At first I thought, *did I just hear that*? I turned around to see an old woman with a scowl on her face glaring right at me.

With my daughter still wailing I said, "Are you kidding me?"

Suddenly *Sa Sa* and Binky appeared and I grabbed them, ready to just walk away, when she replied, "My children never behaved like that."

I stopped, my sweet girl finally calming down as my own temper tantrum was about to start. I took a deep breath, turned back to her and said, "And this is why your children are in therapy trying to figure out why they hate you so much." Then I walked away.

In the background, I heard someone say, "You tell her Mama!"

This is pretty much how I dealt with anyone who attempted to shame me when my kids were having a meltdown in public. I never yelled or screamed or became angry. I just realized I had wit and a way with words and I would use them to shame them right back.

Okay, maybe I should have just walked away, and often I did, but sometimes something needs to be said. Look, here's the sad but honest truth: Your kid is going to lose it, and usually at the worst possible time—in the grocery store, in a restaurant, at your niece's wedding. It's going to happen and guess what? Sometimes you're going to be cool under pressure and sometimes you are going to go ballistic. This is just how it is, and the best way to deal with it is to recognize that you're human, and even though you believe you're totally evolved and mature and will always do the right thing there will be those times when you'll explode like a banshee in defense of your child. You are going to have "bad mommy moments" and say things you might regret a millisecond after they leave your mouth. However, if you can simply take a moment to say to yourself, "Wow, that sucked" and move on, you're going to be thankful later. You can't beat yourself up for wanting to throttle your kids, because the reality is, you are going to feel that way.

By Betsy Chasse and Debbie Spector Weisman

As they get older it's even harder to keep your cool on. Sometimes you're going to scream back, "Are you fucking kidding me?!" Yep, I've done it, a few times. (Well, maybe more than a few times.) But after the storm you will calm down, and for me, that's when I go back to my kid and apologize. We talk it out and most of the time they get it. They see, *wow, mom is human, she's like a real person with feelings.* I've found losing it on occasion is exactly what everyone needs to remember that.

As you can probably tell, a big part of this book is about reminding you that it's all going to be okay and to give yourself a break. No matter how many different books you read or which discipline tactic you use (123 Magic, time outs—or as my kids love to call it—the mad finger) it's not always going to work all of the time. For me I've found that being consistent with my yes and my no is the best discipline tactic I have.

Kids have personalities. They are individuals, and the more you listen to how they listen, the better your discipline will work. Start early! One trick I've learned is that standing above them with

It Came Out of my Vagina! Now What?!

a mad finger doesn't work. Get down to their level, look them in the eye, and then use the mad finger.

A quick side note about pacifiers and blankets and stuffed toys as soothers. I used them with my daughter and until she was about three and half; it was all the rage. Slowly we removed them and everything worked out just fine. It didn't interrupt feeding, it didn't make her teeth all crooked and ultimately for her it worked well. My son, however, couldn't care less. Again this is one of those things you and your child should work out together. Leave the peanut gallery out of it.

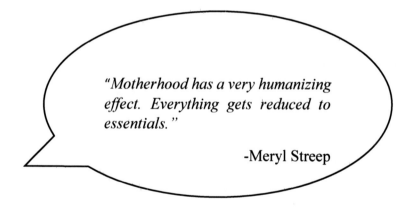

"Motherhood has a very humanizing effect. Everything gets reduced to essentials."

-Meryl Streep

Debbie: My first education on child rearing came from watching *I Love Lucy*. Let me tell you, Lucy made parenting look pretty easy. Little Ricky hardly ever cried, he never demanded much, and he played a mean set of drums, seemingly without ever complaining about practicing. Not only that, but Lucy seemed to always be able to go out with Ethel or get into one of her crazy antics without having to worry about what to do with the baby. There were some times when we actually saw her hand the kid off to Mrs. Trumbull, but for most of the time Little Ricky was the boy who was not seen and not heard.

I thought that's what it would be like to have a baby. Sure, there would be the times I'd need to feed her, change her diaper, and, of course cuddle and love her. But I thought I could spend the rest of my time pretty much doing what I was doing before she was born.

That's why the first meltdown came from me, and not from my baby daughter. I was so clueless as a first-time mother. At the time of her birth, I was writing novels full time, and I had a manuscript due in the first month after she was born. Naively I believed that I could plop her down in her infant seat on the floor next to my desk and have her stay there contently while I typed away. Yes, I know this sounds crazy, but having not been around babies most of my life, I honestly thought taking care of a baby was as simple as that.

It Came Out of my Vagina! Now What?!

Of course it wasn't. Even when I wasn't on a deadline, she squirmed like a worm every time I put her in that seat. I couldn't get mad at her; after all, all she was doing was acting like a baby. Still, I was forced to deal with the issue of how to juggle being a mom and being a professional right off the bat, and I was totally unprepared.

It took a lot of caffeine, time shifting and help from my husband to get that book out. Then I put the writing on hold for a few months until I felt she was old enough for day care, and I could get a few hours to myself.

My other self-inflicted meltdown centered on breastfeeding. I came of age when the shift from formula to breastfeeding was gaining a lot of steam. What that meant was that there were a lot of women out there who were zealots when it came to the breast. They made women who chose to use formula feel like third-class people who ought to have their mothering licenses taken away from them. Being sensitive to this peer pressure, I was anxious to be the best breastfeeding mother in the world.

By Betsy Chasse and Debbie Spector Weisman

Alas, it was not to be. Between my raging hormones and my daughter's inability to suck, I was having a hard time getting my milk to come in. Not that I didn't try. I engaged a breastfeeding consultant who showed me how to pucker the little darling's mouth around my breast to encourage the milk production. When that didn't work, I started wearing this crazy contraption where a formula-filled tube was taped to my nipple so that she'd get nourishment while learning how to suck and trying to push my boobs to production.

This process was not only time-consuming but demoralizing. Nothing I did seemed to work. Finally, when she was three weeks old, I called quits to this breastfeeding boondoggle. I knew I'd be damned to hell by the breastfeeding bigots, but I decided it was more important to love my daughter than to love breastfeeding. I ditched the equipment and went straight to formula feeding.

It was the best decision I could have made. She thrived on formula and grew into a very happy baby, until…

Solid food. Back in the old days, when my babies were little, we were told to start out with cereal and then gradually introduce fruits, vegetables, and finally meats. This meant prepared baby food, and for the most part she loved it. But when it came to meats, you'd have thought I was trying to feed her poison. She'd not only spit out each spoonful I'd shove into her mouth, but she let loose with the loudest, most ear-jarring wails I'd ever heard. I'd manage to get enough into her to satisfy my concerns that she was eating enough protein to survive, but each feeding session with meat became a war of wills, and most of the time she won.

Looking back on those days now, I realize she was just giving me a prediction of what I could expect moving forward. As a young girl, she was the only one in her group who didn't love cheeseburgers. Now, as an adult she never eats meat, except for the occasional chicken, and she's wonderfully healthy.

I recall that both of my children behaved fairly well in public, though I'm willing to admit that my memory of this phase might be analogous to that of childbirth—it's easy to forget the really painful stuff. Once we were inside the safety of our house, however, anything went. In my son's case, the issue was organization. Every day, by the time nightfall came, my house looked like a tornado had run through it. You name it—toys, clothes, empty food wrappers, stray pieces of paper—were all over every room. I'd start out very politely asking him to put his things away, and more often than not I'd be answered with a defiant, "No!" This would be followed by a rant, sometimes ending in a full out body-on-the-floor, hands and feet flailing performance.

I tried all sorts of things to get him to comply. I gave him warnings. I gave him time outs when he refused to comply. I gave him stickers when he did listen. All of this resulted in varying degrees of success.

The one thing that did work all of the time—and I'm ashamed to admit it—is yelling at him. That kid knew how to push my buttons, and at the time I had no other tools in my box to make him behave differently. This is probably not what someone who's reading a book for advice wants to see. But it's the truth. Sometimes the baser human instincts are going to win out. I never hit him and would never have done anything to intentionally traumatize him.

It Came Out of my Vagina! Now What?!

My daughter was guilty of one transgression that I've learned is a pretty common one in many households. When she was around three and blessed to have more toys and playthings than you'd find in the typical Toys "R" Us, we decided she was old enough and mature enough to leave in her room to play by herself. At least that's the reasoning we told ourselves. The truth might have been more along the lines of wanting some adult "us" time, but since that's all in the past we don't have to go there now.

In any event, one day when I'd thought I'd left her to play dress up, I returned to her room to discover she'd redecorated the walls with her entire collection of crayons.

I'd like to say I was incredibly delighted with her toddler masterpiece and enlightened enough to bestow praise for her ability to mix black and yellow in such interesting fashion. But we're being honest here, right? My first reaction wasn't thinking that I was looking at the next Picasso, it was wondering where I was going to find a painter to cover up this mess. In other words, I lost it, she lost it, and the ability to make this a teachable moment was lost forever.

By Betsy Chasse and Debbie Spector Weisman

This is one area of parenting where I'd like a do-over. I made lots of mistakes dealing with discipline and behavior. Some of them were minor and forgotten by all of us. Some left marks that had to be cleaned up when we all were old enough to know better and to be forgiving.

It's not too late for you. Let my mistakes be a guide for you. In the tradition of doing as I say, not as I do, here are my suggestions of what to do when confronted with a meltdown:

1. If you're in a public place, like a restaurant, take your child outside or to a place where you can be alone. You don't want to hear the crying and neither do strangers. Try to be respectful of their space.

2. Let the kid cry it out. If you're home or in a place where this is feasible, this can work.

3. Talk. If your child is old enough to understand, explain why he or she needs to do what you want. Sometimes, all they need is

the feeling that their voice matters, even though in the end it's what you want that really counts.

4. Time out. Physical breaks in the action really do work. It's kind of like pushing a reset button.

5. Have alternatives at hand. A lot of the time, meltdowns are caused by boredom. Providing other ways of keeping your child engaged can often do the trick.

6. Change the scenery. If you're inside, go outside. Outside? Go in.

7. The old saying about it taking a village to raise a child is true. Sometimes you have to ask for help and not be ashamed to admit you need it. It's not always easy to do, and I understand that. But some choice and wise advice from a family member, counselor, spiritual advisor, friend or shaman can go a long way toward creating peace in your family.

By Betsy Chasse and Debbie Spector Weisman

Chapter 7
Tales from the Potty Training and Sleep Wars Sleep Wars.

Betsy: I'm starting to notice a theme. Your kids will tell you how it's gonna go, whether it be potty training or sleep training, disciplining, or eating—I often wondered who was training who here.

Now some moms might disagree with this theory of letting your kids be the guide, and I'm not suggesting you just allow your kids to run rampant all over your house and your life. But I do truly believe that parenting got easier as I chilled out a bit and let my kids help me figure out the best way to go on any particular subject.

Take potty training. Each one of my kids kinda decided when they were ready. For sure my daughter was easier, but eventually both my kids figured out poo-ing in the toilet was a lot easier on everybody.

It Came Out of my Vagina! Now What?!

As a first-time mom, I read all the books, the blogs, talked to other moms, and lived in utter panic that one day I would really screw her up. I'll never forget the time I was worried that my eight-month-old baby wasn't rolling over yet. This was in the heyday of the autism scare and of course I bought into the hype. According to all the books, my child should be rolling over and she wasn't—so I called my mom in a panic after having researched all the signs of autism on the web (seriously sometimes you should just put the Google down!) and explained my concerns.

Mom was silent for a few moments (it seemed like an eternity) and then she said in a very serious, stoic voice, "Betsy, are you sitting down?"

OMG, I thought—this is it. This is where the shoe drops—and she says, "I have to tell you something important..." (long dramatic pause...)

"Elora did not read that book," she told me. It took a minute for that statement to sink in... *Huh... she's right.* My kid had not read all the books outlining at which moment in her life she would roll over, pee in a toilet, sleep through the night, eat organic fair trade veggies (or when she'd get taller than me and roll her eyes in utter disgust...now that would have been helpful).

The reality was my sweet cherub was in fact, cherubic. She was a very healthy baby, i.e., chunky and roly-poly, and damn adorable I might add.

I invite you right now to try something. Put down this book, lie on your stomach and rise up on your arms. Stay there for ten minutes. Yep, I said ten minutes. That is hard, like really hard, *even if you do yoga everyday* hard. This is what it feels like to an eight-month-old baby.

In that moment I stopped running a timer for tummy time, threw out the books and just decided to allow my kid to grow at her own pace. Guess what? She didn't walk until she was fourteen-months old, either. Why would she, when everyone in her life loved nothing more than to hold her and snuggle her and carry her wherever she wanted to go?

For my son it was our family dog that taught him to roll over. Together they created a game that would keep him entertained for long periods of time. He would climb over her body and she would

It Came Out of my Vagina! Now What?!

flip over, thus rolling him over. They did this over and over and over again until he did it on his own. He also walked when he was eight months old, so go figure. I find it ironic how I waited with bated breath for my daughter to take her first steps, and how I tried (unsuccessfully) to keep my son on all fours as long as I could.

There is some really awesome research you should be aware of around brain development and cross-crawling, but if your baby decides to go bipedal before the book says they should, don't fret. Just teach them to dance; they get the same neurological boost!

I had heard the sage old advice, "Get your baby on a schedule." Ha, I say, Ha! Maybe my failure to get my daughter to sleep through the night meant I was a failure at being a mother, but I doubt it. I can laugh at it now, but in the moment, the fact that my daughter woke up just about every hour on the hour until she was almost three was no laughing matter. The memory of many a night sobbing, covered in baby vomit, sleep-deprived and desperate have yet to fade into mommy memory.

Have I mentioned my little angel is willful? (I actually think this is a good thing; now if I could only get her to realize she should be willful to everyone *but* her mother!) Early on I tried everything to get her to sleep, including placing her in her crib with a video baby monitor on and watching her scream and pull herself up by the bars of the crib. Okay seriously, this is probably the most hurtful thing you can do to yourself (probably not to your baby). I sobbed as she sobbed and cracked every time. Running down the hall to scoop her up and bring her into bed with me, where nestled against my breast she slept, for an hour.

One night as I attempted this barbaric form of mommy torture (I swear I should have just performed self-flagellation and moved on), I put my baby in her crib. Miraculously, she lay down all by herself and closed her eyes. *Wow—I did it,* I thought. After several nights of utter misery, it worked! I left the room and thought, *Hey, I can pee.* Then as I came out of the bathroom I thought, *Gee, she's really quiet.* I went to have a peek at the video baby monitor and to my absolute shock and horror, there was my baby dangling head first, holding on for dear life to the other side of the crib, upside down! She had managed to flip herself over the bar and was hanging on precariously, and to my amazement, not making a sound. I can only imagine what was going through her head.

My head was exploding as I ran down the hall to rescue her before it was too late. After that, the super expensive Pottery Barn crib became a toy box and Elora slept with me. So did her brother.

As I write this, my daughter sleeps through the night in her own bed; my son does too, although he still sneaks in on occasion. Sometimes, even now, we have slumber parties and all snuggle up together—and I wouldn't have it any other way.

I have a confession, I read a book about how indigenous women taught their babies to pee and poop on command by making this shhhhh sound, thus eliminating the need for diapers, I thought this was pretty amazing, so for about a week I tried this, every time my baby would pee I would run to the toilet, hold her over and go shhhhh, she thought it was a hilarious game and would giggle and wiggle and then I would end up covered in pee. I just ended up frustrated, smelling of pee and feeling like a failure. So I gave up and bought more diapers, I won't share with you the exact moment my daughter decided to potty train herself, but one day she just did, very matter o'factly…just the way she does most everything.

My son, as I'm told most boys do, took a while. He couldn't care less if he had a wet diaper and much to his chagrin, I'll tell you he wet the bed and sometimes pooped in his pants until he was almost 8. Luckily I was a pretty chill mom by then and I realized getting upset, punishing him or embarrassing him, wasn't going to help either of us. I went out and bought one of those nifty mattress covers and every night before I went to bed I would wake him up. This was often a hilarious experience. Imagine dragging your drunk friend out of a bar, that's what it was like getting my son to the bathroom, but you know what, after a while his body clock got used to it and voila, bed wetting vanished, and the poopy pants, well that eventually stopped too. He and I made a deal, he wouldn't hide it from me (because that was kinda gross, nothing worse than shoving your hand into a pile of laundry and pulling out a little surprise), and I wouldn't get mad, it's his body I told him, he had to listen to it, or smell l really gross. It was his choice and guess what, he figured it out. I still encounter the occasional skid marks, but overall it's pretty fresh in the underwear department.

Kids love learning about the body and how it works and when they realize that their body is communicating with them, they think it's kinda fun. Teaching them to listen to their bodies, to know when they are hungry, tired or have to pee is empowering, but I still announce prior to leaving the house, "Anyone have to pee?"

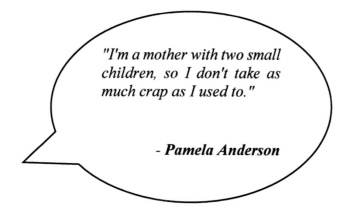

"I'm a mother with two small children, so I don't take as much crap as I used to."

- *Pamela Anderson*

Debbie: Maybe for you it came after you changed the 1001st diaper. Perhaps it happened after the first time. I'm talking about that blessed thought: *I can't wait till this kid's out of diapers.*

It's true. Even after you've gotten to the point of being a pro and are able to do it blindfolded and one-handed, changing diapers is a drag. There's the sticky goo on the butt that always manages to collect under your fingernails no matter how hard you try to avoid it. There's having to wipe every last fleck of poop from the inner crevices around the penis and the inevitable rash that forms even after you're sure you've done everything you could to prevent it.

Then, of course, there's the smell. Oh, the smell! Even with all that modern technology has done to mask that natural aroma with fragrant oils, disinfecting diaper pails and the like, there's no getting around that smell. Yes, it's your kid and you love him or her. But still…you can't wait for the day when little Mona or Chase can use the toilet.

There's just one hitch—getting past that hump of actually teaching them how.

There are plenty of books on the market that give you step-by-step instructions and varying philosophies on how and when to cross this milestone in your child's development, so you won't get that here. What you will get are real, from-the-field war stories on how I survived persuading my little ones to jump over this hurdle.

It Came Out of my Vagina! Now What?!

For instance, I didn't need to read a book to know when it was time to train my daughter. She gave me her own signal, by defiantly ripping off her diaper, time and time again. Usually this happened at the most inopportune times, like when I was in the middle of cooking dinner or just about to leave the house to go to the supermarket. The saving grace was that she only did this in our house. Of course she thought it was the funniest thing, laughing as she did so, totally oblivious to the reality of what cleaning up her mess from the new wall-to-wall carpet meant to her poor, tired, overworked mother.

She was ready. I was ready. I bought one of those tiny little plastic potties, believing that having a special place to pee would give her some sense of entitlement. If memory serves, it also had a bell or some sort of chime on in, so I would literally get a tinkle when she did a tinkle. Clever, huh?

If you met me now, I'd come across as a very patient and caring soul. Well, half a lifetime ago I was anything but. I was so impatient that I eagerly raced out and bought a book about how to potty train your child in one day. I wasn't going to wait around patiently for her sphincter muscles to strengthen. I wanted results and I wanted them now! If the book said it was possible, then by all means I was going for it.

I decided that T-day was going to be on a Saturday, when I had no other commitments and could devote my entire concentration to this project. I had read the book and was ready to do—no pun intended—my duty.

Rule number one for getting what you want from your child? Bribe her! In this case, the reward was candy. (This was way, way before I was enlightened about the effects of sugar on the body, so again, this is one of those *do as I say, not what I do moments.*) Anyway, armed with a bottle of apple juice and a bag of M&Ms, we headed for the bathroom.

Thus began a methodical plan that ran like clockwork for the next few hours. Make her drink some juice, wait for the pee, then give her an M&M when she did the deed. Then more juice, pee and candy. Rinse and repeat.

Believe it or not, it worked! My brilliant daughter latched on to the concept very quickly and by mid-afternoon and a half bag of

It Came Out of my Vagina! Now What?!

M&Ms later, she bought into the system. The potty was her new best friend. She even took to pouring the pee into the big toilet and washing her hands afterwards like it was no big deal.

I think what really cinched it, though, was the final reward: big girl underpants. Even at that age, she was a bit of a fashion maven and knew that pretty pink panties were a big step up from clunky diapers. She understood that if she wanted to wear these dainty garments she'd have to keep them dry, and if she wanted to do that she'd have to use the potty. What a smart kid!

For her the system worked like a charm. She moved seamlessly from toddler in diapers to little girl in panties, and I felt like a genius for getting her there so quickly. The biggest kick came a few days later when my husband and I were sitting in our family room watching TV while she was in her room playing with her toys. The two of us were startled by a strange noise coming from the hallway. It was the sound of a flushing toilet! She did it without being asked, without telling us in advance. Our little girl was growing up!

By Betsy Chasse and Debbie Spector Weisman

When it came to my son, instinctively I knew I had to do things differently. I'm not sure why. Maybe it was just that I knew boys matured differently from girls and that he wouldn't respond to the one-day deal as easily as she had. I somehow knew he'd take longer, even before we got started.

First, we had the issue of the training potty itself. He wanted nothing to do with it. No coaxing, bribing or any amount of M&Ms would get him to go near it. At this point in his young life he'd already been to day care and preschool and had seen his share of "grownup" toilets. To him the potty was something for babies and he wanted nothing to do with it. He was open to the concept of using the toilet, but we had one more roadblock to clear.

My husband and I are both the right size. But to the rest of the world we are considered *vertically challenged*. (By that I don't mean we're little people, we're just on the lower end of the height scale.) When we first got married and considered the possibility of children, we joked a lot about breeding for shortness. We never stopped to really consider the effect this would have on our offspring. They'd be short, too, and have to deal with the same challenges we'd had.

In my son's case, that was the toilet. Since he refused to use the potty we had no choice but to train him to use the toilet, but being the size he was at the time that meant he was too short to reach the bowl. If he got on his tippy toes he could manage to hit the water in the bowl with his stream, but I realized that wasn't realistically going to work in the long run.

This is where it paid to be married to a guy who's handy with tools. Understanding the situation right away, my husband went out to the garage and quickly fabricated a platform to put in front of the toilet. This created the height my son needed for a perfect shot into the toilet. When he saw what he could do in this position, he was hooked! Standing and squirting was a lot more fun that peeing into a diaper. He also responded well to all that "You're a big boy now" talk that went with his being able to use *his* platform to do his business.

Even so, it was still a bit of hit and miss with him, and it took a week or two before going to the bathroom was second nature to him.

But the main point is this. They're all going to get the hang of it eventually.

Chapter 8
Baby Envy

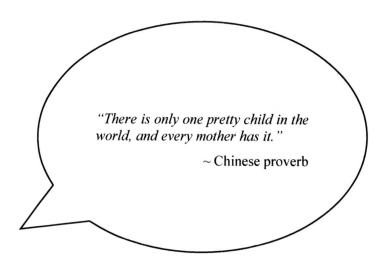

"There is only one pretty child in the world, and every mother has it."

~ Chinese proverb

Betsy: Okay, listen. It's time to get real. There will be moments throughout your parenting life when you are going to compare yourself to other moms and your kids to other kids. It's perfectly normal, and even if I tell you not to, you're going to do it anyway. It's human nature: the grass is always greener, the stroller is always better and the other mom's baby is behaving oh so much better than yours is right now. But shhhhhhh…here's a secret. Just as much as you are wondering, *how'd she do that?* Just as much as you're oohing and ahhing at her mommy prowess, chances are she's doing exactly the same thing.

Yep, humans are funny like that, and not just about our parenting skills. We spend a lot of time worrying about what everybody else thinks of us and comparing ourselves to them, when the reality is that they don't have time to worry about you because they are too busy worrying about what you're thinking about them. Oh, what a paradox!

Woman are known to be catty, gossipy and downright bitchy, but I beg to differ. Most women are actually very lovely and if you do wonder, *hey how'd she do that*, then ask her! I know. Crazy, right? Wouldn't you love to have another mom ask you about how you got your kid to eat that green veggie or how you got them to leave the park without a full-throttle melt down? And mom peers (moms with kids the same age as yours) are usually on top of what's going down with the whole parenting thing because they are right there in it. Plus, as a bonus, you might find someone who finally gets you!

It Came Out of my Vagina! Now What?!

You will, on occasion, find that mom who thinks her kid's shit doesn't stink and parades around all June Cleaver-like. Well, let her. Just talk smack about her when she's not there. (Okay, I'm kidding.) Sadly, she's probably the most insecure one in the bunch. If you can't break her with a few self-deprecating war stories about vomit between your boobs or a baby poop stain on your blouse when you went to work, then I say let her go. There is only so much you can do. Your life is way too busy and you have much more important things to do than to deal with someone who can't face their own overstuffed dirty diaper pail. (I am going to run out of baby puns here soon!)

If you're stuck with her—say she's was in the mommy club before you got there, she runs the mommy club or she's your sister—well then learn to just grin and ignore her. The cool thing about snobby mommies is that they can only annoy you if you let them. Eventually other newbie moms join the group and Ms. Snobby and her friends inevitably turn their attention to the fresh bait.

By Betsy Chasse and Debbie Spector Weisman

There are times when I think it's important to step in and say something. I was living in the woods of Washington State when my first child was born and the mommy club pickings were slim. But we had a good group. We were all New Age hippies and the parenting style was, shall we say, loose. We had a more free-roam style and tried often to let our kids explore and learn for themselves. Safe to say there was not a helicopter parent in sight, which I thought was a good thing. Most of us moms kept a close eye from a short distance and employed the "distract and detour" method as opposed to the screaming *"Johnny get the F#CK over here"* method.

There was one mom, however, who took this concept a bit too far, refusing to ever say no to her child, like as in *never*. One day as we were playing on the trampoline, her little guy decided that throwing a small wooden train at the heads of the other children looked like fun. Throw one earned the warning: "Honey that's not a wise choice," from the mommy to her three-year-old. After throw two Mommy laughed, "Oh honey, now don't you want to do something else?" to which he replied "No!" At this point I'm

It Came Out of my Vagina! Now What?!

thinking, *well he knows the word no…so?* Uh-uh. No dice. Throw three hits my daughter squarely in the face, at which point I walk up to the little sprite, snatch that wooden train from his grip, look him in the eye and say, "No! We do not throw things at people!"

The kid looks back at me, and for a moment I thought, *Uh-oh this kid's gonna lose it.*

To my surprise, not a peep from the boy. Instead, I hear a sharp gasp from the mother. "We don't use that word!" To which I replied, "Well, he did, so clearly he gets it."

As we turn to face our children again, we find that the little tyke has put down the train and is happily jumping on the trampoline. What a concept-- use it for what it's for.

The mom tried to shame me for disciplining her son. Luckily a few of the other moms jumped in to my defense. I stated that while I agree that constantly telling our kids no was just going to teach them how to tune it out, sometimes a strategically placed "NO!" goes a long way.

Most importantly when it comes to your mommy tribe, take your time in finding one that works. You're going to spend a lot of time with these women, so pick them wisely and remember that a no is sometimes better than a yes.

> "Always remember your kid's name. Always remember where you put your kid. Don't let your kid drive until their feet can reach the pedals. Use the right size diapers... for yourself. And, when in doubt, make funny faces."
>
> -Amy Poehler

Debbie: This is especially true when dealing with a particularly special category: the mother who constantly crows about her child's developmental achievements. This phase runs through the first two-and-a-half years of a child's life, encompassing everything from the moment your child goes from being a cute lump of breathing flesh, and continues until he or she is a real life human being with a brain. There isn't a mother out there who isn't monitoring all the growth milestones, and secretly—or not so secretly—comparing her child to his or her peers.

When you treat this as a game, it's a harmless conversation to undertake while watching your kids pour sand over each other at the park. But because they're human, some mothers take this too seriously and are either too smug when their child rises above the milestone or too traumatized when their kid is on the short end of the stick.

I have a very good friend who managed to give birth to a large baby. There was nothing wrong with him, but because he was so large, he had more difficulty than most in doing the things that all babies do, such as rolling over and crawling. He didn't walk until he was nearly eighteen months old.

My friend was smart. She trusted her instincts that he was just fine. Her doctor also assured her that her child was physically normal and mentally alert. This enabled her to tune out all those other mothers—and there were quite a few, I should say, including some of her own relatives—who were convinced that something was amiss. However, if she hadn't had that inner resolve, she could have easily gone to pieces.

My own mother went through this with me. I was bald until I was three years old. All my baby pictures reveal a hairless baby who often looked like a cue ball in a dress. She could have seethed at the sight of cute little babies with thick shocks of hair on their heads. But she knew that in time, I'd grow my own.

That's the key here. In the end, all of these milestone comparisons mean nothing. My friend's son grew into a very handsome, very successful adult. His body shape made him a natural for football and being on his high school team boosted his popularity and self-esteem. So what if it took him longer to be ready to walk in cleats? I not only grew hair, but had such a thick head of curls that as an adult, I used to have to have my hair thinned.

I actually lost a good friend over the issue of mom envy. One of my friends became obsessed with writing her annual Christmas newsletter, but in my opinion she took it a step too far. In her world, there was nothing her kids couldn't achieve. You would have thought *best* was part of their name, as in: "Petey wrote the best poem in third grade" or "Lily was the best athlete in her class." If they awarded GPA's of 6.0, her kids would have earned them. It became almost sickening to read about their achievements. My kids were great, but they could never reach the pinnacles of these two. No one could.

After three or four years of reading about these impossible accomplishments, the only way to get away from this hyperbole was to cross her off my mailing list.

In today's world there's a new platform for mom envy: social media. It's natural for moms to post photos of their kids, and most people enjoy seeing them. But it's the mom who posts five times a day and is obsessed over how many likes she gets that has to be avoided. Getting those photos in your news feed is almost as obnoxious as those incessant cat videos. When she goes overboard like that, she's not posting to be proud; she's demanding the attention to make you believe that she's special and deserves to be awarded Mother of the Year.

By Betsy Chasse and Debbie Spector Weisman

My number one piece of advice for dealing with the overachieving mom can be summed up in one word: perspective. Keep a healthy skepticism about anything this woman crows about. Chances are, her need to brag about the unique specialness of her offspring stems from her own fears and self-doubts. Don't be cowed by her. Instead feel sorry for her. She's so insecure she needs to live vicariously through her kids. You, on the other hand, have it all together. You don't care that your kid's not the smartest, best looking, tallest, most athletic, most artistic or any other most you can think of. You're fine with mediocrity because it's your kid and you love him and that's all that matters.

It Came Out of my Vagina! Now What?!

Chapter 9
Mom Envy

"When it came time for me to be blessed with the natural wonder of motherhood, I too thought, "I got this!" I was raised by Super Vi! I am a full time realtor. A career that affords me to work out of the house, create my own hours, take my child with me. I am golden! I got this! So I thought...until one day when my beautiful baby who used to sleep for 3 hour naps and I could get so much work done, decided she was done napping at 2 years old and would rather scream constantly in the back ground while I was trying to negotiate million dollar properties. Laundry was never my thing and suddenly the piles I used to make fun of from other moms were an envy.

At least they were able to keep it all in a pile for crimany sake. I was just happy to find matching socks.... Then school started and wow, game changer. Not only am I racing against the clock every morning, my daughter is lucky if I remembered to get fresh milk for her cereal and have baggies in the house to put her 1000th Nutella sandwich in. I am lucky if I have a clean shirt on let alone a shower. Make up? Hahaha.

~ Janie Mahon Mom of 1

Debbie: Here's a sad but hard truth. There's always going to be someone better than you in every group. Whether it's your mommy and me gathering, church congregation, or school organization, *someone's* going to have it put together more than you. Her kids will be wearing trendy togs, immaculately tailored with not a food stain in sight. Their hair will be fashionably shaped

By Betsy Chasse and Debbie Spector Weisman

by the best children's stylist in town. She'll strut them around in the most trend-setting stroller or gently guide them while they master that $500 tricycle. She'll have made sure they were bilingual from birth and will be hell-bent on making sure they've earned their black belts by age eight. They'll be tutored from preschool on and genetically programmed to get nothing less than an A minus on their report cards.

There's only one way to deal with a mother like this: avoid her. Maybe that's the coward's way out, but if you're a woman dealing with the daily stresses of raising a child, working outside the home and striving to keep a healthy relationship with your husband, it's an honest response. You're flat out way too busy to devote precious mental energy on ways to keep up with or to outdo the woman who seemingly has it all. Don't even go there.

On the other hand, there's one place where comparisons are going to be inevitable and there's no getting around it. I'm talking about the birthday party. This is where the Supermom pulls out all the stops, and where a gathering with cake and juice simply doesn't cut it any more.

It Came Out of my Vagina! Now What?!

The overindulgence of the birthday party is a phenomenon that has crept up, little by little, over the years. Back in ancient times, when I was a kid, these were simple gatherings. The moms dropped off the kids at the honoree's house, where a dozen or so kids played simple games like *Pin the Tail on the Donkey* or *Duck, Duck, Goose*, or *Tag*. This was followed by the appearance of the birthday cake, the obligatory singing of *Happy Birthday*, and the opening of the presents. Party over.

By the time my kids were of party age, the typical home celebration included the arrival of a costumed character who would play games and entertain the kids while the parents stood in the background, drinking white wine. The food was more elaborate, though still simple things like pizza or hot dogs, followed by a custom-made birthday cake that was coordinated with the theme of the party. My son's favorite party, for instance, was headlined by Batman, who swooped into the room swishing his cape over my son's face, and delighted the crowd with more bat puns than I ever thought existed.

By Betsy Chasse and Debbie Spector Weisman

Alas, I took the themed character party a little too far. I made the fatal mistake of inviting Bart Simpson to my daughter's eighth birthday party, realizing too late that the pre-packaged party banter was too young for these pre-tween's sophisticated tastes. It took her six months to forgive me.

Even so, I firmly held to my belief that it's crazy to go overboard on kids' parties. Some years I went outside and held the parties at bowling alleys, gymnastic centers, and pizza parlors. Yes, I had a party at Chuck E. Cheese's and survived it. I kept the event focused on the birthday girl or boy and didn't give a second thought to all the things I didn't do. For instance, one of my friends held her son's party at Dodger Stadium. I couldn't compete with that, and didn't even try.

I realize that today the parties can get pretty complicated, with bouncy castles, pony rides, laser tag, face painting, magicians, batting cages, spa treatments—sometimes all of them at once. Then there are the issues I never had to deal with: Does the food contain peanuts? Is the cake gluten-free? Have I invited every single person in the class? Have I done everything I can not to offend anyone?

Believe it or not, I never had to deal with those issues. Peanut allergies were virtually non-existent a generation ago. While I respect those who have adopted a gluten-free diet, I have a feeling that many are just jumping on the holistic bandwagon and really don't have celiac disease. Yet now their desires have to be taken into consideration when dealing with the party issue. And, frankly—at least in the circles I traveled in—no one was keeping tabs on who was invited to which party. I'm sure feathers were ruffled, and I imagine there were parties where my kids were left off the invitation list, but we all survived. Today things are different, and everyone is striving to be inclusive, which means you have to carefully monitor your invitation list.

My take on all this is pretty simple. Do what you can. If you have the means to throw a party with all the bells and whistles, by all means do so. Your kid will definitely love you for it. But don't do it just because the neighbor down the street did the same thing, especially if it means you'll be eating mac and cheese at home for the next two months to make up for it.

You don't need a bankroll the size of Canada just to show your peers how much you love your child by financing a party that's beyond your means. In fact, with a little imagination and planning you can stage a spectacular DIY party on a budget. I'm not a party planner and I'm not going to regale you with tips here, but there are plenty of online sites that present fine ideas for parties for all ages of children. Your kid may rant and rave if the party isn't as slick and flashy as the one thrown by the woman who has it all. But if you put in the effort, your kid will secretly know you care. Of course, it may take *years* before he or she admits that they appreciated your efforts, but that comes with the territory of parenting.

> *Motherhood is so sentimentalised and romanticised in our culture. It's practically against the law to say there are moments in the day when you hate your children. Everyone actually has those moments.*
>
> -Barbara Kingsolver

It Came Out of my Vagina! Now What?!

Betsy: As my daughter first entered school I felt it was important to look my best when dropping her off. In the early stages, you have to actually get out of your car and walk them into school, which means seeing—and being seen by-- other moms and teachers Appearing as if you have it all together seemed important at the time.

Every morning I would get up, shower, and put on something hip and cool, but not too cool; I didn't want to look as if I was *trying* to look awesome, I wanted to look like I *was* awesome naturally and without any effort. This was easier when we lived in the country; a clean pair of sweat pants without coffee stains would do.

But then I moved to the city, and as my daughter entered her first day of big city school I'm sure she had butterflies, and so did I. As we walked up to school that morning, the realization that my clean sweat pants would not do sunk in. A sea of moms in business suits and flashy jeans, complete with all the right accessories and lipstick, passed us by.

By Betsy Chasse and Debbie Spector Weisman

There was a beautiful park close to our house, and when we first moved to the big city I took my kids there in hopes of meeting up with some local moms and kids and to begin building my new tribe. My daughter quickly found a friend in the sand box and as our children played, the other girl's mom approached. *Wow, perfect in every way.* Slick but casual going-to-the-park outfit? Check. Hair in a "I just threw this together" pony tail, but still freshly dyed and cut? Check. Nails (both mani and pedi, naturally) perfectly colored and looking gorgeous in her not-bought-at-Rite Aid flip flops? Check.

I felt way out of my league. Cool for sure, but a bit hippie for this neighborhood. I had a moment where I wanted to wave a magic wand and trade in my sweat pants for a pair of skinny jeans, but then I had a moment of clarity. *If I don't pre-judge this woman, maybe she won't prejudge me.*

We began to chat. I explained that we had just moved back to California and told her what school we would be attending. Her eyes brightened as she said, "Oh we'll be there too!" We figured out our daughters would be in the same grade. I began to feel relief after seeing that while she was for sure more together fashionably than I was, she was nice and easygoing. With our park time coming to a close, I gathered up my kids as my new mom friend reached for her purse. "Keep in touch over the summer," she said as she handed me what I thought was going to be a business card.

Ha! That was no business card; it was, in fact, a mom card. Yep, a mom card. I can barely manage to keep a pen in my purse and here she was with a cute little pink mom card with all of her kids names on it, her name and phone number. *Impressive for a mom of three girls*, I thought. Quickly I ran home to order my own and to pick up some new jeans, get my nails done and cut and dye my *we just spent all our money moving and I've been using store bought* blonde hair.

Not only did that mom have cards, she had color-coded, dated file boxes containing all of her children's artwork, hand prints and pictures. She had even edited and organized every video she'd ever taken of her three little darlings. My keepsakes consisted of a big plastic bin with everything thrown in, including the videos and pictures. What?! File according to age and date? Yeah, right.

By Betsy Chasse and Debbie Spector Weisman

There will always be a mom you think is doing it better than you. As I said in the chapter on baby envy, you can't avoid feeling inadequate as a mother at least once in your mommy life. It's inevitable. Mommy guilt is the most common sickness among moms; we excel at making ourselves feel "less than" because we excel at comparing ourselves to others. So STOP IT! I mean, what else can I say except: *you're awesome.* Believe it.

After about a month of getting up every morning a half-hour early just to primp and look my best for the walk to school I realized, *you know what? This isn't me.* I'm a comfy-sweatpants-in-the-morning kind of gal. If I have somewhere to go after drop off, sure, but really I do not need to impress anyone, except myself and my kids.

On the day of that realization, I put on my Target sweatpants and a T-shirt (coffee stained and all) and we walked to school. I kid you not, that morning as we approached the gate, I saw the supermom coming from the other end of the block. Her hair was wild, her baby was on her hip, a crying two-year-old was in tow and her school-aged daughter was running for the gate. And she was dressed in...sweatpants! As we met, she looked at me. I could see she felt embarrassed, so I looked at her, smiled, pointed to my coffee stain and said, "It's one of those kind of mornings." We laughed together. We actually became good friends. She is still always more organized than I am and I appreciate that about her. I am always more relaxed than she is and she appreciates that about me.

You can only do what you can do. If you want to do more, then do it. If you don't, then don't. I have often rebelled against this notion that we must find balance and that somehow translates into going to a spa, or out with the girls. Here's the thing: when you have kids, sometimes you're not going to have time for that. I mean, scheduling the time, finding the babysitter and then leaving your kids for three hours can be stressful. By the time you get to where you're supposed to relax, you're so stressed out that it takes you the entire three hours just to settle in—and then it's time to come home!

Balance is a perspective. Supermom is a perspective. You have the power to choose what that perspective looks like, what works for you. I decided early on to have the perspective that I already am a super-balanced mom.

Chapter 10
Teamwork, or How to Survive Being a Sports Mom

Betsy: I have a friend that I never get to see unless we cross paths on the soccer field. Why do I never get to see this friend? Because every day—I'm not kidding, every day—she is busy driving her kids to something. Soccer practice, basketball practice, dance class, singing class—you name it, they're doing it. The poor mom is exhausted. Not only does she work full time outside the home, but after work she is essentially a chauffeur. Not to mention being stressed out by the financing of all those classes. I'm exhausted just thinking about it, and I can't imagine how the kids deal with it. To be fair, her kids seem to enjoy it, so who am I to judge.

One thing for sure is that as your kids get older and into school, they are going to have lots and lots of homework (this is a huge pet peeve of mine, so don't get me started). I think it's important to be reasonable with your expectations about all the extra-curricular activities you schedule for your kids.

Here's my philosophy: one activity per season, and if they fall in love with it, then they stick with it until they don't. Try to schedule each kid's activities on a different day and nothing on at least one day of the weekend. Most importantly try to find things close to home and things their other friends are doing. This comes in handy for carpooling and saves you from losing your mind driving all over town, eating in the car and trying to get homework in besides.

Early on, say around age five or six, let them start trying things—and don't go all gender specific either. Your daughter may love sports and your son may love ballet. Let them find what they love and give them time to figure it out. This may not be easy to do, but do it anyway. As a parent it was hard for me to let *them* do the finding, but I did. My son has learned to love football and I'm now dealing with to tackle or not to tackle. I think I'm going to error on the side of caution; he might be annoyed with me now, but I know he'll forget about it soon enough.

It Came Out of my Vagina! Now What?!

My daughter loves music and art and decided early on she doesn't want to do the shows, perform on stage or be in the band; she loves creating on her own and I honor that. Giving them the power to choose is a great way for them to learn about themselves; they might learn how not to be good at something or to they might find something they are good at…even better, they can learn how to become good at something, even when it's hard. But most importantly it gives them a sense of control in their own lives. Most of their lives at the moment are up to mom and dad, so giving them a sense of choice gives them a sense of empowerment and responsibility.

Some advice I was given and I'm happy to give back to you now is that when your kids find something they love; it helps them make better choices when they get older. They figure out that if they get bad grades or get into people or things that don't support their favorite pastime, they lose it. This is probably the most important life lesson I think a kid could learn.

Debbie: When I first thought about dealing with the sports mom, the picture in my mind was the mother who needs to take charge of the team. Never mind that there's a coach or some other figure who's actually guiding the kids on the field, she's the one who's convinced her child is always in the right. She's the one that's yelling the loudest at the ref or the umpire that her kid got wronged in some way.

We already tackled the idea of the supermom; a lot of her negative tendencies show up in the sports mom as well. I'm just going to let it stand that you just have to accept that there's at least one woman like this in any team situation. Let her rant and rave. Feel a little pity for her, as you realize that this game might be the highlight of her day and she has no other outlet for expression.

That brings up another aspect of having your child play in team sports: expectations. The whole idea of having your child play on a team is grounded in some valid concepts. It's important for him or her to get exercise and be physically fit, and an organized sports event provides that opportunity. Playing on a team also instills the idea of discipline. Becoming a good player requires learning the rules and working those muscles so she can throw a ball more than 12 inches in front of her. That's not going to happen the first time she picks up a ball, so she has to practice. It's not easy to get a child to practice, but if she's on a team and has others around her who are trying to do the same thing, she'll tend to be more motivated.

Sports also instill responsibility. If you're on a team, the others are expecting you to show up—and if you don't, there are all sorts of consequences. Your child may have to incur the wrath of his teammates who'll get upset if he's not there to play goalie on the soccer team. Or by not showing up, he'll miss the after-game pizza party. Repeated absences will result in him getting kicked off the team entirely, as those poor overworked and underappreciated coaches don't like it when they're caught shorthanded at games.

Now here's where expectations come in, and by that I mean *your* expectations. You may have loved playing soccer as a kid and have looked forward to seeing your offspring head-butting on the field ever since you bought her that cute little size 12-month soccer onesie with matching striped socks. How are you going to feel when you march her to practice on that first day and find her kicking and screaming—not at the ball, but at you for forcing her there? Are you going to be the kind of mom who's going to insist she stay on the field? Or are you going to accept her desire not to mess it up with cleats?

This is one of the toughest crossroads one faces when being a mom. It's that day when you realize that your little one has a mind of her own, desires of her own and opinions of her own. In my experience, nothing is gained by insisting she be on a team if she doesn't want to be there. Chances are she'll end up sitting on the sidelines, bored out of her mind and counting the minutes till the game is over and she's allowed to go home.

The truth is, you'll go through a bit of a mourning process as you say goodbye to the dream you had in your head of seeing the team proudly prance around the field with your son in the air after he kicked the winning goal. Some things are just not meant to be. But that's okay as you know you love him anyway.

I was never on a sports team, since my mom had a big thing about my not getting dirty and it's hard playing field hockey in a dress. But I'm a big baseball fan and I longed to see my kids play Little League. My daughter, being a girlie girl, had no interest in it

It Came Out of my Vagina! Now What?!

at all, but I had hopes for my son, who didn't seem to mind when I put a giant plastic bat in his hands when he was three.

At age five, I marched him down to the local baseball field and signed him up for T-ball. As I've said earlier, our family is a bit height-challenged and it was no surprise that he was the smallest kid of the bunch. Even at the tightest setting his cap settled down over his ears. I thought he looked so cute. But cute isn't what playing T-ball is all about. As much as he tried, even I had to see that he was never going to grow up to be the next Alex Rodriguez. It hurt to come to that realization, and my writing this now is probably the first time he'll learn about this. (There are just some things you don't say to a five-year-old.) He managed to get through the season, but I was smart enough to realize his athletic talents lay elsewhere.

I'm a big believer in involving your child in some sort of physical activity, so we experimented with other sports. He played soccer for a few years and liked it, but he really found his passion with flag football. He played on his school team all the way through elementary school and later found success as a high school wrestler.

My daughter, on the other hand, never had much interest in team sports. She loved gymnastics, though, so I encouraged her through several years of flips and parallel bars and balance beam. She also spent time running on a track team, which was sort of a hybrid between team and individual sports. She was on a team, but doing events on her own. As long as she wasn't sitting home all day talking on the telephone—one of her other pastimes—I was happy.

In short, here are my tips on how to be the sports supermom in your family:

1. Be realistic #1. Playing sports is supposed to be fun. If you force your kid into something she doesn't like, nobody wins. Hopefully by this point in her life you've developed an idea of where her interests lie.

2. Be realistic #2. Every mom wants to think her kid is a superstar and is destined to win an athletic scholarship to Notre Dame or even a career in the NFL. Fuhgeddaboudit. Get your kid playing sports because you want him to be fit, make friends, learn about teamwork, and all that good stuff talked about earlier. Don't get into the mindset that his athletic prowess is going to be your meal ticket into your golden years. This is for his sake, not yours.

3. Okay, this isn't really a bullet point, but I'm reminded of one of my pet peeves—those participation ribbons or trophies that are awarded to everyone on a team. Yes, it's nice to be recognized for being on a team. But playing sports can also be a learning experience for what lies ahead in life. When you grow up you don't get a trophy for participating. You get paid well or win awards for being the best. It should be the same in youth sports. The kid who scores the most should get special recognition. I don't buy into this philosophy that there are no winners and losers. Real life doesn't work that way.

4. Participate. The opposite of that mom who lords over the spectators is the mom who either drops her kid off and leaves or the one who never signs up to take snacks. Teamwork extends to the parents as well.

5. Don't over participate. If the approved snack list calls for oranges and fruit bars, then provide that to the team. Don't show up with sushi platters or buffalo wings you've heated up in your portable stove.

6. Make sports a family activity. Everyone—Dad, siblings, even the family dog if allowed—should attend the games. It's a great bonding experience. Some of my happiest memories are hanging out at the all-day track meets, where we brought a cooler, folding beach chairs, a blanket, and pitched a sun canopy. As a bonus, we got to hang out with our neighbors and others in the community.

Chapter 11
Wait, This Isn't My Sweet, Obedient Child! What Happens When Your Kids Hit the Pre-Teen Years and the Hormones Start Kicking In

> "...do everything in moderation", she said. This was one thing my mom told me early on and whenever I feel myself going too far or too guilty or too much of anything I always hear that in the back of my head.""
> ~ Erica, Debbie's grown-up daughter

Debbie: The biggest shock of my young parenting life came one day when I accidentally walked into my daughter's room. The first shock actually came from her, who didn't at all like it that I, her mom, was invading her privacy. Not that I was doing it intentionally. I'd just done the wash and was absentmindedly doing what I thought was the right thing by taking her freshly folded clothes into her room. I hadn't even realized she was in there, that's how stuck in my own head I was. She looked up with me with that upset glare that only a daughter can have for her mother. *What are you doing here and why won't you leave me alone?* She didn't actually say those words, but my mother radar, now turned on, could read the message loud and clear.

I, on the other hand, was having a hard time getting my brain to adjust to what I was seeing before me. My daughter was in the middle of changing her clothes, and I came face to face with a new visual. Her flat chest had erupted into two tiny mounds.

This can't be true, I thought. She's just a little kid! She's too young for boobs. What happened to my little baby? She's growing up way too fast.

I should add here that I never had this moment with my son. He was way too private to allow me to see him naked after the age of three.

But that's what little bodies do, and there's no getting away from biology. In fact, studies show that children reach puberty at a much earlier age than they used to. The average age today for girls is between eight and thirteen, for boys, nine to fifteen. These ranges are a full year earlier than they were only twenty years ago.

All those statistics are well and good, but they don't do anything to really prepare you for the day when you see evidence of bodily development on your child. This is really the moment you have to take a deep breath and realize they really are growing to maturity and it won't be long till they're packing up and moving out on their own.

Once those hormones start kicking in, there's really nothing you can do but be a good guide and a loving shoulder to cry on for your child. They're seeing these changes in their bodies too, and despite any videos they are shown in school or books you read them at home, they're confused and full of questions. What do I do with that hair on my legs and what is that stuff that's growing *down there*?

There's no bigger shock in a young girl's life than the day she wakes up and sees blood in her pee. If you're a smart mom, you've already educated her in the simple fact that it's the start of her period. But there's a big gap between reading about it and actually experiencing it. Depending on your child she'll feel any or all of these emotions: embarrassment, excitement, curiosity, anger, fear. One thing she probably won't be feeling is delight. I don't know any girl who's loved getting her period. I mean, be honest here. I'm willing to bet that one of the great things you enjoyed about your pregnancy was *not* having your period. You know what I mean.

Here's my take on how to handle modern day periods. We've come a long, long way in sanitary pad technology. By the way, did you know the expression *being on the rag* came from the days women had no choice but to stuff rags in their panties to sop up the flow? I remember the days when I had to strap on a really thick pad that was connected to a belt I wore around my waist. You can bet I felt like I died and went to heaven when they invented stick-on pads. (Actually by that time I had graduated to tampons, but that's another story.)

In the past few years there's even been a trend among environmentally conscious women to wear reusable cloth menstrual pads. They come in all sizes, from panty liners to maxi-pads, and are meant to be machine washable. Advocates say they're more comfortable, reduce chafing, are chemical-free, and of course, are good for the environment as they reduce landfill needs. If you're fine with using them, I say god bless you, and I applaud your decision. But as with disposable diapers, I'm just not enlightened enough to ever want to use them myself.

Another relatively new development is the menstrual cup that fits inside the vagina. Some claim they are safer than tampons, but they have to be cleaned after each use—which can be a pain for people like me who are slaves to convenience.

In short, it's no fun being an adult and having to deal with that monthly madness. I started my daughter with pads and allowed her to determine her menstrual destiny after that. I figured it was her body and the time was coming to start letting her make her own decisions.

Seeing your own child entering that first step to adulthood is scary. Those raging hormones have a natural outlet and that's a four-letter word spelled B-O-Y-S.

That means one thing. It's time for The Talk.

By Betsy Chasse and Debbie Spector Weisman

If you're smart, you've dropped hints about the birds and the bees all through childhood. There are quite a few books on the market that speak about how the body works in ways that are both easy to understand and comforting to children. There are way too many to mention here. I suggest you hit Amazon.com to find those that resonate with you. If you've read any of these to your child or given them to him or her to read, then the typical response to the suggestion of, "Hey, sweetie, I think we need to talk about boys/girls," is going to be answered with, "Aw, Mom. I know all about that."

Trust me, they don't. They might think they do, from the "truth" they get from their friends or something they pick up from the internet. But, really, they're clueless. The first time they actually deal with someone in a boyfriend/girlfriend kind of way they're thrown into a whole new world. They'll expect to need to look and act cool about it too, which just adds extra pressure. This is where you're going to have to be strong and be ready to answer all those same questions that were running through your brain when you were that age.

It Came Out of my Vagina! Now What?!

Now for the good news. If you've been a loving parent up to this point—if you've been the kind of mother who's always there for her son or daughter, who's always willing to listen, who's not quick to make judgments, who's always been supportive—you'll do just fine.

Here's something that helps a lot: rules. When kids start to get into their tweens, they're itching to rebel and to keep stretching their boundaries as far as you'll let them. They'll demand their freedom and will be arrogant enough to believe they actually know better than you.

Don't give in to their delusions. They may now tower over you in height, but you're still the parent. You have not only the power but the right to set the standards under which they live. You decide when they're old enough to date. You decide how late they can stay out with friends. You decide what places may be off-limits, what language or dress may be inappropriate in public, whether or not they can get a tattoo or whatever else they're demanding.

They'll protest. They'll yell and scream and call you names you never imagined hearing from that little infant you brought home from the hospital. You'll get upset and hurt and maybe even second-guess your decisions. Don't. Secretly—and believe me they will never admit it in public—they'll appreciate these guidelines and limits you set for them. Without them they're clueless or they'll be forced by peer pressure to do something they might not really want to do. Being able to say, "My mom won't let me," may be the most beneficial words to them at this age.

> "And when she one day turns on me and calls me a Bitch in front of Hollister, Give me the strength, Lord, to yank her directly into a cab in front of her friends, For I will not have that Shit. I will not have it"
>
> -Tina Fey – Bossy Pants

Betsy: I have to be honest (okay when have I not been in this book!) My kids have never been totally obedient, and the truth is, I wouldn't have it any other way. I have tried to teach my kids to question everything, to use their own brilliant minds and think for themselves. I realize now I probably should have qualified that with "except when it comes to anything I say." You know: question everything, except your mother!

Oops…oh well. I've got spirited, rebellious kids who have an opinion (hmm, sound familiar, Mom?) But here's the thing. Somehow my kids know when and where they can express this anarchy and when they should probably smile and play the sweet angelic child role. So far it's working. I guess most people are fooled.

My daughter is eleven as I write this book, and she embraced the pre-teen *I'm going to be pissed off at you until I'm thirty* part of growing up with a vengeance. I've been told by friends that this is actually a good thing, although as I'm standing in my kitchen deep breathing after yet another "I hate you and I hate my life" moment, I'm having a hard time believing that. I don't recall doing this at eleven. But science is saying, and she is living proof, that kids are growing up faster and faster. Hold on young mamas, because who knows, if right now eleven is the new thirteen, then lordy are you in for it!

By Betsy Chasse and Debbie Spector Weisman

As I'm driving my kids to something one day, I'm only half listening as my daughter prattles on about who has a crush on who, who's got hair on their legs and who needs to start using deodorant, all I can wonder is, *Wow, I'm here already; wow that was quick.* The conversation turns to what middle school she will be going to and that the school in my neighborhood has uniforms. I try to explain that most middle schools have uniforms, and that most middle schools are trying to alleviate the hormonal distractions middle schoolers go through by making sure they are dressed appropriately, you know, no shoulders showing, no crop tops that show their midriffs. (Of course to me this makes no sense, because a teenage boy could get a hard-on with the shifting of the wind, but hey, I'm reaching here. Anything to try and help her see her next educational phase as something to look forward to.)

I can tell the emotions are ramping up, because a pre-teen girl's emotions change faster than a teenager changes into different clothes a block from the house when Mom's not looking. But I'm off my game and I'm like, *seriously kid, this is nothing.* I said to her, "Look, wearing a uniform is not going to kill you." She looked at me, stunned into a brief moment of silence (very brief), her big blue eyes welling up with tears. In her best Scarlet O'Hara voice she said, "Yes! Yes! Yes! Mother it *will* kill me!"

You know what? I laughed.

Yep...Mommy failure 101. Never laugh at your pre-teen's emotional breakdowns over clothes, her favorite pencil being chewed or misplaced friendship bracelet—really it could be anything. The important thing to remember as a mom is to not laugh.

This is really hard by the way, so practice while you can. In my defense I have about 34 years on her, and if I'm honest, it took me almost 30 of those years to learn not to ball up in a corner sobbing with snot running into my mouth about the most mundane of things. Why on earth would I expect her not to do the same?

After I laughed, I realized my mistake. She sobbed uncontrollably in the car saying over and over, "You don't understand. You've never had to deal with this."

All I could think of was, *oh honey, this is nothing, wait until you find out one of your best friends made out with your boyfriend.*

By Betsy Chasse and Debbie Spector Weisman

The shit is really going to hit the fan then! (Luckily that didn't come flying out of my mouth; I do have some restraint). No, in that moment I saw that for her, this truly was the end of the world. *Her* world. She hasn't had 45 years of heartbreak and disappointment, she's only eleven. I've got a whole lot more practice in the art of recovery, of discernment, of figuring out what really was worth the all-night ice cream binge, sobbing in the bathroom on the floor in mismatched pj's. For her this was big. If I was going to help her understand that it wasn't big, I'd have to first show her I understood how big, to her, it was.

It's interesting how many of the tricks we use on our toddlers actually work on our kids as they grow. When my daughter was three or five I always tried to get down to her level, especially when I needed to communicate something she didn't want to hear, like the word no.

The exact same theory applies to your pre-teen. I've learned that most kids do not realize until they are much *much* older, that you were, in fact, eleven at some point, too. They picture you as you are, old and wearing really ugly pants and uncool, oversized tops. They have no point of reference. Of course they think you have no idea what they are going through, because to them you have never done it.

Well, seeing is believing! Out came the pictures of me when I was eleven and I hated my year book picture, when I was sixteen and had a laughably crazy hairstyle, and so on. More importantly (listen closely here…) I had to learn to listen first and wait for the right moment to share any wisdom. Because it seems pre-teen (and onward into teen-hood) kids don't want wisdom. They want understanding, they want acceptance, they want someone in this world to just love them. They feel like everyone in this world is trying to teach them and you're the last person they want that from. Ironic, I know. But it's true. It was the hardest truth for me to accept. It's not about being their friend, but it's also about not "being their mom." It's about being their guide, which is very different.

I struggled with this in the early stages of rebellion, but as I practice the art of shutting up and allowing her to speak, to share, to express, I see her relax. I see her soften and oddly enough when I do speak, she listens.

Chapter 12
The Battle of the Bulge…or Yes, You Can Get That Bikini Body Back

> *"After 3 kids I feel like an old balloon! Don't know what I mean…take a new balloon blow it up and release. Doing it once you'll see the difference, do it 3 times? Now you get what I'm talking about. One of my lovely kids told me I had beautiful long boobs….they obviously agree with my analogy. Got to love their honesty."*
>
> ~ Michelle Murry Sterns – Mom of 3

Debbie: If you read the earlier chapter about childbirth, you know that my hormones were screwed up when I had my kids. But I wouldn't be surprised if you didn't know that, if you rushed to this chapter as soon as you opened the book. I mean, why not? You can admit it. Who wouldn't want to know the latest and greatest secrets on how to shed all that post-pregnancy weight? I sure would.

Well, now I feel a little bit like those internet ads that promise the *Great Revelation Into the Untold Mysterious Method For Guaranteed Weight Loss*. Sorry, ladies. There's no big secret here. Yes, that chapter title is misleading. It says you can get your bikini body back. That much is true. There are ways to shed weight that work. But if you didn't have a bikini body to begin with, all bets are off.

Anyway, those screwy hormones were my way out of losing weight. During my first pregnancy I gained about thirty-five pounds, and on me that was a massive 35% weight gain. My face was three times its normal size and about half of that was the result of the massive amount of acne and female beard hair that decided to make my face its home for the duration.

I thought all of that would change after the baby was born. Uh-uh. A week later I had zits the size of small states on my nose and hair growing in places it never should. My doctor, being a doctor, thought this needed further investigation. Being a specialist, he referred me to another specialist, an endocrinologist.

On first examination this doctor thought I might have a tumor on my adrenal gland. In a way, I was lucky. If I'd been born a generation earlier that would have meant cutting me open for exploratory surgery to see if his hunch was right. Fortunately, there was ultrasound and all those pretty pictures of my insides turned up negative. Whew, no tumor.

Still, there was no explanation for all this negative stuff going on in my body. All we could do was take a wait-and-see attitude. If things didn't change, further tests might be necessary and then who knows what.

But a good thing was happening. That first week I lost a good eight pounds or so. That weight loss continued at a steady rate and by the time my daughter was six weeks old, I was back to my old pre-pregnancy weight. It took a few more months for the zits to decrease and electrolysis got rid of all that beard hair.

By Betsy Chasse and Debbie Spector Weisman

Therefore, my secret method of weight loss is to have bad hormones. Yes, I know that's not an answer, so I'll try to get a little more sensible here.

There were a couple of other things I did at the same time that also could have contributed to the weight loss. First off, I felt really great after I gave birth and went back to exercising three weeks later. Now I know that most people say that's too early, but I went back to the gym with no ill effects. The gym I went to at the time also had a mommy-and-me workout, and being able to hang with my baby and stretch and bend at the same time was a real plus. She liked it too. My husband was also accommodating in watching her so I could go to regular aerobics classes, too. Since we all know that exercising is a key element in weight loss, I have to give these workouts some credit.

The other thing I did was watched what I ate. Now, I admit this was a new concept for me. My pre-pregnancy diet often consisted of lunches of Diet Coke and popcorn, and as soon as I learned I was pregnant I knew that wasn't going to cut it any longer. I made an effort to eat reasonably healthy food when I was pregnant and continued that trend (at least for a little while) after I gave birth.

Between regular trips to the gym and cutting the chocolate chip brownies out of my diet, I managed to keep my weight exactly where I wanted it until I got pregnant again. In fact, I still have a photo of me in a bikini, taken when my daughter was about eighteen months old, which shows me being in the best shape of my life.

Then I decided to get pregnant again. I gained about twenty-six pounds when pregnant with my son, and again, hormones helped me lose all my weight gain postpartum. This time, however, the reason for my weight loss was my thyroid. I won't get into all the medical details here but in short, I went through a period of rapid weight loss that was followed by a period where my thyroid stopped working at all. I would have blown up like a pumpkin at that point, except that my doctor implored me to eat a totally no-fat, no-carbohydrate diet. This kept the weight off until I was put on medication to control my thyroid function. From then on I managed to stay in a pretty decent weight range where I never weighed more than ten pounds above my pre-pregnancy weight. That lasted pretty much until menopause kicked in, and that's the subject of another book so we'll stop here.

To summarize, here are those "secret" tips to losing that post baby flab:

1. Eat regularly. One of the worst habits, especially when dealing with the unpredictability of a newborn, is to eat on the run or make your own eating needs an afterthought. Your baby needs you and you've got to take care of yourself. Eat three meals a day. It helps if you can plan ahead and have meals you can easily assemble or heat up.

2. Ditch the evil snacks. When you don't eat regularly, your tendency is to want to snack, and we all know it's so much easier to pick up a cookie than cut apart an apple. If you do feel the need to snack, make sure your refrigerator is stocked with healthy eats, like fruits and veggies, which are not only good and tasty for you, but good for your baby too.

3. Make friends with exercise. As soon as you're physically able, get your body moving as much as you can. Take part in an organized class at a gym, go to a yoga studio or take long walks in the neighborhood with your baby. Don't stay seated for more than thirty minutes at a time. Keep moving.

4. Decide you want to lose the weight. You may say you want to lose five pounds, and at the same time reach for another dish of ice cream. You can't have both, so just decide which is more important to you. Then be okay with that choice.

5. Find a diet buddy. Chances are you have a friend with a newborn that also wants to lose some weight. Be each other's support system. Having someone cheering you on or helping to keep you on track will go a long way toward getting you to your dieting goal.

6. Relax. Stress is a major impediment to weight loss because it causes you to produce a hormone called cortisol that tells your

body to keep all those fat cells. Of course being a new mother is going to be stressful, and I realize that telling you to chill out might result in making you feel even more stress. All I'm going to say here is to try to de-stress if you can. Listen to a guided meditation, go on a long walk, or take a bubble bath with lavender water if you can.

7. Did I say relax? Our culture makes us want to think that there's something wrong with you if you don't have a picture perfect body. But let's face it. The truth is that most people don't. Have you ever seen before and after photos of celebrities, for instance? Their pictures are photoshopped, airbrushed, and filtered to make all their imperfections disappear. They may also look great walking down the red carpet, but underneath all those beautiful gowns are yards and yards of Spandex and other materials that compress the flesh into a pleasing shape. Or they pay a small fortune to personal trainers who monitor their exercises like drill sergeants, and to personal chefs who prepare every diet-loving calorie they consume. Either way,

it's a false image and it's not like you and me. Don't buy into it.

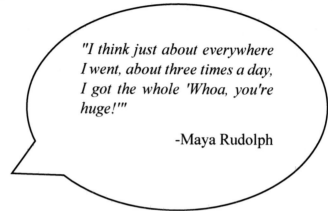

"*I think just about everywhere I went, about three times a day, I got the whole 'Whoa, you're huge!'*"
-Maya Rudolph

Betsy: The best thing you can do for yourself is to be happy with your mind and your body. If you're really determined to lose weight, you'll make that commitment and do all that you can to make it happen. If losing weight isn't all that important to you, that's okay too. Remember that golden rule: A happy mother makes a happy baby.

Let's face it, everybody is focused on the "body after baby watch" almost more than they are on the baby bump watch. Tabloids are abundant on the newsstands and screaming with headlines such as *LOOK AT HER BODY JUST 2 DAYS AFTER GIVING BIRTH!* It's enough to make a woman want to crawl under her Boppy and hide for the next year or so. Why a year or so? Because that's what it should take a normal woman to get her "bikini body" back. Of course, like my cohort in all things mommy, Debbie says the first part is to have actually had a bikini body to begin with.

Humans are so obsessed with how much we gain during pregnancy and how fast we can lose it after the baby is born; it should become a new Olympic sport.

With my first baby I was on that endless treadmill. I wasn't super skinny pre-pregnancy, but I was petite and had a nice flat bikini tummy I was proud of. About four months into my pregnancy it was a full-fledged baby bump, and I was enjoying one of the only perks of pregnancy I could find—eating just about whatever I wanted.

Yep I gained weight, a lot of it. I was checked for gestational diabetes and given just about every test there was, but there was nothing wrong with me. I was just feeding a very hungry baby who was born at a whopping nine pounds, and perfectly healthy I might add.

It Came Out of my Vagina! Now What?!

People were not only focused on my weight, but also on my daughter's weight. At three months she was the size of a six-month-old. But you know what? She was healthy and happy. I told the pediatrician to stop comparing my baby to their charts and just make sure she was healthy. Seriously, why start her weight complex before she's even out of diapers?

I breastfed and that helped me drop weight at a normal pace. I did work out, but I had to wait three months so I could heal from my C-section. My working out was more about getting my core strength back and less about having a perfect body. The truth is, I just didn't care. I was a busy working new mom and that was pressure enough.

Our obsession with women's bodies isn't anything new. We've gone from buxom and bodacious to skinny Minnie and back again. I swear I can't keep up and neither should you.

When I was pregnant with my son I was literally asked like 1000 times, "Are you having twins?" Are you serious? Again, I had to drink the Kool-Aid and starve myself so I could be tested for gestational diabetes and once again gave birth to a perfectly healthy baby, this time a ten-pound seven-ounce baby boy. He won the award in the hospital for the biggest baby born that week!

I have struggled with my body image for as long as I can remember, and after having my second child something happened. I stopped. I didn't stop caring about my health, I just stopped trying to fit into someone else's bikini. In the chapter about feeding baby, I shared how I fed my kids healthy food and snacks, which meant their diet was my diet. I did mommy-and-me yoga, walked a lot, and used exercise more as a meditation and less with the goal of losing weight.

Here's what I can tell you about losing weight. Diets usually don't work. That's probably something you've heard a million times. You've seen people go on diets, lose a bunch of weight and then gain it all back again. It happens all the time.

Then there's another truth. After you have a baby, your body behaves differently than it did when your diet consisted of Diet Cokes and Cheese Whiz. Even if you had healthy eating habits pre-baby, your body just performed something miraculous and grew a whole other being inside of it. If that doesn't change your chemistry, well then, maybe you're not human. Your hormones are finding their way back to normal and your metabolism is figuring out it doesn't need to feed two beings anymore. There's a whole lotta changing goin' on in there, and your body needs time to figure that shit out. Give yourself the time. Don't go starting some crazy shake diet, or start eating only kale. Eat a healthy diet and let your body get back into harmony.

The other thing about fad diets is that the brain isn't buying it. Your brain is a pretty awesome piece of machinery, and it knows you better than you know yourself. You can trick it for a while; you can trick your chemistry and drop the weight, but the reason it usually sneaks back on is because your brain doesn't believe you when you say things like, "I want to look like Cindy Crawford in the 80's." Because you probably don't.

If you do, then great—go for it. But be realistic with yourself. There is no reason you can't have the body you had before baby, but don't kill yourself trying to get it. I found that pacing myself was everything. I discovered that in a little over a year after each pregnancy my body found its way back to a very happy place. A balance of exercise, eating right and an abundance of baby play time did the trick.

Chapter 13
What to Do with All Those Pictures?

Debbie: You don't want to miss one precious second of your child's life. Thanks to today's technology, it's easy to create a history of her life. Perhaps too easy.

I'll bet it started when you were pregnant. At least once a week—if not more often—you took selfies of your tummy to track the increasing size of that little bundle growing inside you. After the birth, you kept taking photos. You with the baby. Your husband with the baby. The grandparents with the baby. Friends with the baby. The baby by himself.

You keep taking pictures until the memory in your smartphone fills up. Only then do you remember to download the photos to your computer or to the cloud. Then you start the process all over again.

At this rate you'll have a fantastic collection of every move this kid ever makes.

By Betsy Chasse and Debbie Spector Weisman

Now do the math. Let's say you snap ten photos a day, every day. That's seventy photos a week and 3640 photos in a year. At that rate, by the time he's ten you'll have 36,400 photos of the kid. That doesn't even take into consideration special occasions like birthdays, holidays, sporting events, trips to the zoo, vacations and such, where the kid-to-picture ratio expands exponentially.

However, you look at it, that's a lot of pictures.

The sheer volume creates some practical problems. Let's say you're visiting your Aunt Patty, who wants to see snapshots of baby Serena. You can't wait to show her that cute shot you took the other day of her eating spaghetti and getting it all over her face. You whip out your phone and you both get bored to tears as you valiantly swipe past the out of focus shots, the off-kilter shots, and the ugly expression shots until you come to the ones you're looking for. Or perhaps you forgot you just had to do a memory dump and now have no way of showing her anything.

At this point you're probably thinking, *I'm going to post all the good photos online and then they'll be available for everybody to see.*

It Came Out of my Vagina! Now What?!

Here's where we take the reality test. Really? Okay, I'll admit this much. At first you'll be posting photos as fast as you take them. You're proud of your child and you'll want everybody to see him on as many platforms you have. But take it from me, the novelty will wear off after a while, especially as you notice the number of likes you get drops with each successive posting. Your friends may love you and enjoy seeing snaps of little Liam, but they're too kind to admit that every day is too much. The overload may even make some of your more casual friends scroll past your name quickly whenever it pops up on their newsfeed.

When it comes to posting your baby, less is more. People will stop to look at the monthly growth spurts of your infant, and you'll soon see that the once a month schedule works out pretty nicely for all concerned. As your baby grows and gets to be more of a handful, you might also find yourself less motivated to take the time to go online. That doesn't mean you're going to stop taking pictures, though.

Then there's the question of how to save all those digital files. Yes, you can easily store these photos on the cloud, but only up to

By Betsy Chasse and Debbie Spector Weisman

a point. Most basic storage plans give you 5-20 gigabytes of storage which, depending on the size of each individual file, will enable you to save anywhere from a couple of hundred to a couple of thousand pictures. That may be enough to hold you for the first year, but then what? Sure, you can spend more money for more storage, but how much money are you willing to pay for photos that, when you really, really think about it, you might not ever look at again?

One thing you can do is go back and edit your photos and throw out all those not-quite-good-enough images. But, come on, who are we kidding? No one has time for that.

My solution? The flash drive. For about twenty bucks—and even less if you shop around—you can get a 32 gigabyte drive that, again depending on the size of your files, can hold from 4,000 to around 23,000 photos. Fill that thing up, put it in your safe deposit box, and you'll have a permanent record you'll be proud to keep.

Now that takes care of the storage issue. The more pressing issue is how to show off those digital files. In the old days it was a lot simpler. We used to use this ancient stuff called film—that's how your parents took pictures of you when you were little. You'd take pictures until the entire roll of film was shot, anywhere from twelve to thirty six images. Then you'd get them developed and they'd come back in a little folder along with the negatives. By flipping through the photos *that you could actually hold in your hands,* you could decide which ones to copy or enlarge.

It's not always easy with a digital file to be able to tell how the picture is going to look enlarged to an 8 x 10 print. Sometimes a picture that looks fine on a phone has more of a soft focus when it's blown up. Other imperfections may also be easily overlooked in the smaller format. Sometimes you just have to take that leap of fate and trust that what looks good small will look equally good in a larger size.

If you're technically savvy you can transfer your photos to your computer and look at them on a monitor, where all those perfections and imperfections will be much more visible. If you're really handy you can load the photos into a photo enhancing program and really make them shine.

By Betsy Chasse and Debbie Spector Weisman

However, if you don't know the difference between lossy and lossless and don't know how to create a bokeh effect, all is not lost. You can get fairly inexpensive enlargements at many local retail stores like Target, Wal-Mart and Walgreens. There are also lots of online sites that will send you prints and will also turn your photos into coffee table quality photo books. A good rule of thumb is that money will buy you anything.

Now for my practical advice. First I'd better start out with this declaimer. I have two medium sized storage boxes full of photos—many still in their development envelopes—pictures of my kids from birth through their late teens. I always thought that someday I'd take the time to sort through them, arrange them, pick out the best and put them in a photo book, or some other clever way of making them a more memorable memory.

Naturally, if I'd done that, I'd have told you already. Same holds true for the thousands of digital photos I've taken in more recent years. They're stored on my computer and on flash drives. The only times I've really looked through them were for special occasions, the videos we had created for my daughter's Bat

It Came Out of my Vagina! Now What?!

Mitzvah, my son's Bar Mitzvah and then my daughter's wedding. I did a mad search, looking for the best moments of their youth to transfer to photo montages. Then as soon as the photos were used, they got thrown back into the boxes, unsorted and unorganized as ever. The only thing I did have the presence of mind to do was to jot the years the photos were shot on the backs of the prints. At least with digital photos, that information always stays with them; years from now you won't have to guess whether that shot was from Cecil's seventh or eighth birthday party.

This is another instance where my mantra is: do as I say, not as I do. What I'm now going to ask you to do will take some time and effort on your part. But here's where the "do as I say" comes into play. If you do this now, you'll be thanking me when your hair is gray and you want to show your grandkids what mommy or daddy looked like when they were kids.

Here goes. Once a year—my recommendation is the day after your kid's birthday—schedule time with yourself to go through photos taken the previous year. Give yourself a time limit of two

By Betsy Chasse and Debbie Spector Weisman

hours. This isn't something that should take all day to do, and giving yourself a limit will force you to make decisions.

Pick out no more than twelve photos. They don't have to be from each month of the year, but it's a good representative number. Make sure they show your kid in different poses, some close-ups, some activity shots, and some shots with family and friends. Then get them developed into 5 x 7 prints and display them in a photo album. Make 8 x 10 copies of the ones you like the best and they can go in frames that can hang in your hallway, on your night table or on your office desk.

Then the following year, do the same thing. Again, the next year. If you do this diligently, by the time little Fredericka graduates college, you'll have created a family heirloom that everyone will cherish.

But, hey, if you don't, there's always that box of flash drives…

"I know how to do anything - I'm a Mom." - Roseanne Barr

Betsy: Remember my friend, you know the one with the mommy cards, as I said this woman edits each of her videos and pictures after every event and basically every month. Okay, I seriously hate her right now, but in the most awestruck, isn't she amazing kind of way. I literally have drives and videos (remember the little mini-tapes) of my kids and I regret having not gone through them. If you have the time do it. If you don't save them, at some point your kid will have a blast scrolling through the multitudes of pictures you took.

The funniest thing about my kids and pictures is that I have hundreds of my daughter printed. My son came farther in the digital age, and he would often wonder if I ever took pictures of him at all. Here's my solution. At the end of each year I make a calendar for the next year with my favorite pics from that year, and I give them each one for Christmas. They actually love them and keep them in their rooms. It's sort of like a yearbook for the family. They love grabbing one from a couple of years back and my heart smiles when I walk past their rooms and see them looking at them. Kids love memories and this small little book, with not even 1% of the pictures I took of them, helps them feel loved and special. It also keeps me sane, through out the year when I take a picture I particularly love I save it in my calendar file, and right after Thanksgiving I create the book. It's fun for me and they love it.

Chapter 14
Yes, It's Time to Have Sex

> *"If you doubt the reality of a sixth sense start having sex anytime night or day and your child will knock on the bedroom door. Guaranteed."*
>
> ~ Wendy Keown Mom of 2

Debbie: It's two o'clock in the morning. You're getting back into bed after having just fed and diapered your infant daughter. You pull the covers around you, hoping you'll be able to fall asleep and get a few hours under your belt before her whimpering cries force you out of your slumber. Just before you drift off, you turn and face that lump fast asleep next to you. With a snicker you remember the days when you used to use this very same bed for hot and sweaty sex. You wonder when you'll do that again. Then in the next breath you ask yourself, "Will I ever want to have sex again?"

The answer is yes. Childbirth does terrible things to your body and it takes time to recover. Nature manages to wipe those sex urges out of you to enable your genitals to get back to some semblance of normal. It's sort of like nature telling you that now is the time for you to bond with your baby. Your husband can wait.

Chances are your husband understands this. If he's the same lovable dork you fell in love with, he's going to be patient and not force you into doing the nasty till you're ready for it. Remember, he's falling in love with that little child too, and he doesn't want to do anything to upset the other person who helped create it.

Those early weeks after the birth are a time for new connections. You and your husband are figuring out what it now means to be a family. Love is definitely in the air. But love doesn't always have to lead to sex.

That time will come. Allow your body to recover. If you've had a vaginal birth with no episiotomy, you'll be good to go as early as two weeks after the birth. Earlier than that could cause damage as you're still probably having some bleeding and are at risk of infection. If you've had an episiotomy or a C-section, don't even think about it till at least six weeks have gone by.

These are just medical guidelines. You're a woman and you know that emotions are everything. You might not be ready so soon. Your libido is likely not to kick in as soon as you're physically able. For every woman that feeling comes at a different time. One month. Two months. Four months. If you've gone a year without wanting sex, well then that might mean that something serious is going on and you'll need to seek expert advice on why you're avoiding your spouse.

But we're going on the assumption that you're a normal woman adjusting to life as a normal new mom. Here are some things to consider as you get ready to get intimate with your honey once again:

1. It's gonna hurt. At least at first. Your vagina is still super tender, so treat it with the kindness it deserves. If you've never used it pre-pregnancy, now is the time to discover lube. This

gooey product is about to become your best friend, as it will make everything—and by everything you know what I'm talking about—glide in smoothly. Lubes come in three main types: water-based, oil-based, and silicone-based. Water-based lubes are generally the best all-around choice but experiment with what works best for you.

2. It's gonna feel different. Your vagina might not be that tight little thing it was before the baby stretched it all out of shape. Trust me, it will get back to normal, but how long that takes depends on genetics and whether you gave birth to a little peanut or someone the size of the right tackle for the New England Patriots.

3. Birth control. Contrary to old wives' tales, you can get pregnant soon after you give birth. If you don't plan on having Irish twins, don't have unprotected sex.

4. Your breasts have changed. All that new milk in your breasts not only makes them bigger but also makes them feel different too. The squeezing of your breasts that your husband used to

do to turn you on might flat out hurt you now. You may also feel squeamish about his sucking the same breasts that now may be the sole source of nourishment for your baby. This may take some sorting out, but being aware that this could be a potential problem enables you to talk it over with your partner beforehand.

5. There's another delicate breast problem that may crop up. Some women discover they may spray milk while having an orgasm. If that does happen to you, have fun with it. Your hubby may discover he likes it.

   And while we're on the subject…

6. Your orgasms have changed. All those new hormones swirling around your body can have an effect on how you climax. What worked before may not work now. How it felt before may feel different now. Accept it for what it is and be glad you can orgasm at all! After all, a good feeling is a good feeling, even if it's a different good feeling from before.

7. You may fall asleep during sex. You want it. You really *really* want it. But you haven't had a good night's sleep in months. Your body might just say no when your libido wants to say yes. Again, accept it. In a few weeks, the baby will be sleeping through the night and your sleep patterns will return to a semblance of what they used to be.

8. Your husband may have changed. You're the one whose body went through pregnancy and childbirth. You experienced it, but your husband was there too, watching. He may be hesitant to touch you, fearful that he may hurt you or cause you pain. Here's where you're going to have to be the one to lead. Let him know how you feel and when you're ready to do what you know he really wants to do.

9. You may experience *sextus interruptus*. It happens all the time. You finally feel ready for sex and have pulled out all the stops: a sexy nightie, scented candles, soft music, maybe even a sex

toy or two. You're going at it at a furious pace with your partner and feel ever so close to that magical point...and then the baby cries. Being the good mother you are, you feel pulled to rush to her side. Yet the memory of what-might-have-been will linger in the air. Hopefully, though, your patient husband will take care of you upon your return. That's what love's all about.

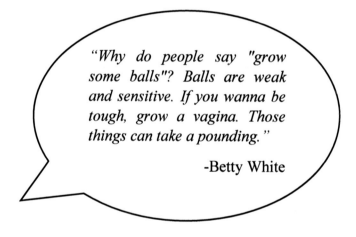

"Why do people say "grow some balls"? Balls are weak and sensitive. If you wanna be tough, grow a vagina. Those things can take a pounding."
-Betty White

Betsy: Let's talk about sex, baby! Ha I said sex and baby in the same sentence! Debbie has it right, for the most part sex was the last thing on my mind for a couple of months after bringing home baby. Especially since mine first didn't sleep, and recovering from a C-section sort of puts a damper on things.

By Betsy Chasse and Debbie Spector Weisman

Face it, everything is weird right about now, the boobs are bigger--that's a bonus--but they don't really enjoy being squeezed and well, they probably leak...ooh sexy! The Vajay Jay is all out of whack and for the most part, choosing between sleep and cunnilingus, well you're going to choose sleep. That's just the god's honest truth, and it's totally cool.

It's absolutely true that men and women are different when it comes to the whole sex thing, but hopefully, you've married the right guy (or at least chosen the right baby daddy) and he's going to be patient. Instead of focusing on the naughty, focus on the connection. About two to three months after baby (I know that sounds like forever, but it's going to go by quick) has arrived start to make time for you and that man to spend quality time together WITHOUT YOUR BABY! (What?!) Yes... really, prepare a bottle, get someone to watch them and go out of the house, even if it's only for an hour or two, start slow, and by about six to eight months, you'll be back to having those uber romantic, super sensual date nights. It isn't just about you and him ya know, it's also about your baby. Allowing your baby to learn to feel safe with your chosen care giver will help them later when you really need a break.

Everyone needs a little me time and so does your baby. This helped tremendously when, around the time my daughter was 24 months and I was ready to wean her, I went away for two days and came back to a happy, fully weaned baby who loved her baby sitter and missed her mommy. We all appreciated what we had and we were all grateful for a change up in the routine. You want an independent kid? The give them some independence, even when they are babies. You're a smart mom, you're not going to have mommy dearest as your baby sitter and I promise you'll be glad you taught yourself early on that it's ok to leave them for a little bit, they will figure this out faster than you will.

By Betsy Chasse and Debbie Spector Weisman

Chapter 15
How to Avoid Mommy Guilt

Debbie: I ought to be in jail…or at least I should have been in jail. I'm guilty of having once left my sleeping baby in the car while I ran into the supermarket to pick up a few items. (I'm not going to say which one it was so they don't have this to hang over my head for the next "Mom has ruined my life" argument.) What I did is a bad thing, and I don't advocate anyone leaving their kid in the car. In fact, years after this incident, my company even produced a public service announcement warning young moms not to leave their child in a car, NOT EVEN FOR A MINUTE.

Yet here I was, guilty of doing what I said specifically not to do. I'm not proud of it. That I'm writing about it now, many years later, shows what a bad, bad imprint it had on my consciousness. But here's the other fact that also needs to be acknowledged: NOTHING HAPPENED.

When I shut the car door on my kid, he or she (see I'm not giving away who it was) was sleeping comfortably in his or her federally approved car seat, and I just didn't have the heart to wake the little darling up for what I knew was going to be a short trip. Was this laziness on my part? To a degree, yes. Wait, what am I saying? It was most definitely laziness. It was also an admission that I was away from my house, and I had visions of this kid not going back to sleep and screaming all the way home. No mother wants to hear her baby cry, especially when you're trapped in a car with no way to relieve that poor kid's agony.

That's why I left my baby in the car. I was certainly relieved to come back with my two full grocery bags and see that my child sleeping just as wonderfully as when I'd left. See, nothing happened.

Uh…that's not exactly true either. While I'm convinced my kid really didn't suffer any lasting damage from this excursion, I sure did. During the ride back I kept replaying alternate scenes in my head. What if someone had broken into the car and kidnapped my child? What if spit up remnants of lunch caused baby to choke on its own vomit? What if a giant tornado appeared and swooped up the car in its vortex? What if the car heated up to 200 degrees

By Betsy Chasse and Debbie Spector Weisman

and burnt it to a crisp? What if my son or daughter woke up, saw I was gone and was forever haunted with the trauma of abandonment? The *what ifs* mounted in my head till I entered my driveway. I was convinced I was first in line for the Worst Mother of the Year award. What was I thinking?

For years, I kept this awful mommy sin to myself. In fact, this is the first time I'm admitting it publicly, and by saying it right now I deserve all the scorn and contempt this confession will heap on me. Short of something really sick and evil, this is close to being the most venal mommy transgression of all.

For a long time after that, I kept replaying this incident in my head. What was I thinking? Am I really that selfish that I put my own sense of comfort ahead of my kid's? Yes, I was guilty as charged, and though I never faced the long hand of the law, I did pay for this in my own troubled mind. I vowed over and over never to make that mistake again. Guilt is a very powerful tool. It worked, and my kids were never again left untended.

Dear mothers, I'm writing this now as a warning to you. Please, don't ever leave your child alone in a car. Not so much for your kid's sake; 99.99 percent of the time nothing bad will ever happen. But for your sake. Mommy guilt is real and will eat you up alive. So don't go there. Ever. Suck it up and do the right thing. Your own conscience will forever thank you.

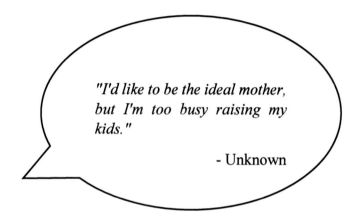

"I'd like to be the ideal mother, but I'm too busy raising my kids."

- Unknown

Betsy: There's not a lot more I can say on this subject without feeling repetitive, I will admit to uttering the "F" word more times than I should, and utterly losing it with my kids, I have spanked and cursed and fallen to my knees on more than one occasion. You will too, and it's totally normal. You will try anything to get that baby to sleep, you will feed them McDonalds and hide the evidence, and you will lose your shit in the most inopportune moment. We all have, and any mom who pretends they haven't been is lying. YOU WILL MAKE MISTAKES.

By Betsy Chasse and Debbie Spector Weisman

Over and over again. I often say to my kids… "If I didn't screw up what will you tell your therapist in your 30's?" Forgive yourself, you've got 18 years, 6 thousand 5 hundred and 70 days until they probably move out of the house (This by no means indicates your mommy days are over) but pace yourself!

Chapter 16
Letting Go

I'd like to take a moment to chat about gender roles. I have a son and a daughter, and from the time when they were little they embraced their gender. You could hand my son a stick and he'd make a gun (even though I never let him play with toy guns and still don't, it seems to be in their genes), and when my daughter was two she rebelled against the cute little comfy pants outfits I bought her, demanding I buy her dresses. Even so, I still have the pictures of my son dressed up in a princess outfit playing dress up with his sister. This is what happens when you have a big sister. Eventually he didn't want to wear a dress. He wanted a prince suit, and bless Grandma for making him one. Embrace boy he did.

During Kindergarten his class had a crazy hair day. My son wanted pink hair, and of course I obliged. We arrived at school and oohed and ahhed at all the fun and crazy hair styles, my son wearing his pink Mohawk with pride.

By Betsy Chasse and Debbie Spector Weisman

One of the moms said to me, "Oh, your son has pink hair. My husband would never let that happen."

I replied in my politically liberal way, "I don't mind what color he has," and kissed my son goodbye.

I knew, of course, what she meant. That somehow, my son wearing pink hair indicated that he might be, well, gay. On the surface, I contemplated, I have no issue with my son or my daughter being gay or straight or ambidextrous or whatever, as long as they are happy. I suspect many parents feel the same way. But since I am one of those "dig deep into the recesses of my beliefs" kind of person, I spent the day considering the idea of having a gay child.

To be completely honest I had to say I would prefer they weren't. Not because of why you might think. The first reason is because that I want my kids to be happy and never suffer or feel unloved— and while we are moving in the direction of accepting that people are different, our world is still often unkind to those that don't fit into our paradigm of puritan thinking.

It Came Out of my Vagina! Now What?!

But the other reason was more intimate, deeply-rooted story that had probably been created that first moment as a young girl when I began to dream of being a mom. Our life is a series of stories we first tell ourselves, and then we go in search of living them. This is exactly what happens when we first learn we're pregnant. All those stories come flooding into our hearts and dreams. We dream of the outfits we'll dress our babies in, we dream of their first day of school, their first T-ball game and everything before, after and in between. Even the most conscious and aware of us do this. We have little fantasies about their weddings and who'll they'll fall in love with. Most of this happens subconsciously and everything is all peaches and pie until something happens that wasn't in the story we created.

I don't know of anybody who doesn't imagine having a perfectly normal, happy child. What happens if that child ends up being gay or autistic or otherwise different from the "normal," and those dreams come crashing down? We get sad. We get angry. We go into denial. We grieve. Then we accept.

By Betsy Chasse and Debbie Spector Weisman

What I found was that from the moment my son was just a tiny sperm in search of an egg I had dreamt up a whole story about how his life would go, his first steps, his first time on a bike, his first bruise or scrape, his first kiss, his first love, his wedding and eventually my own grandchild, I had literally lived his whole life and had grown very attached to it in my head. Because that is what we humans do, we make up stories in our heads and we become very very attached to them, so attached that when our children are born we work extremely hard to fulfil that dream, sometimes at the risk of missing out on who are children really are, gay, straight, silly or serious, good at academics or maybe more of an artist, often whatever we are or what we've dreamed up for them is what we push on them, without even realizing it.

In that moment, when my son was just a wee 5-year-old I saw that I had to let my story of him go so that I could allow him to create the story of his life on his own. This was one of the hardest moments in being a mom, that moment when you know that they have their own lives, their own destinies, their own experience to create and your job is to guide them, not to mold them. That was a

It Came Out of my Vagina! Now What?!

big shift in perspective for me, because often we think of parenting as molding our children into model citizens, perfect people we can be proud of and I what they need is to be loved for who they are. We all know this instinctively, but putting it into action is one of the hardest things you'll do as a mom.

There are literally hundreds of letting go moments, when they first walk, letting them go from your arms, watching them take off on a bike, letting go of the back of the seat, their first day of school, watching them walk into that classroom without you, but this letting go is much deeper than that, it's not about them, it's about you letting go of your version of the story and enjoying watching them become who they choose to be.

"It's not easy being a mother. If it were easy, fathers would do it." - *The Golden Girls*

Debbie: The word that comes to mind when I think about what Betsy writes here is *expectations*. Of course we have plans in our heads for the ideal child that comes out of our vagina—or our womb directly in the case of C-sections. We have that image in our

By Betsy Chasse and Debbie Spector Weisman

heads from…whenever. For some women, that ideal child has been in their minds since their doll-playing days. For others, it comes during pregnancy. We have lots of expectations of how it's meant to be. Which means, of course, a lot of disappointment if you have no way of letting those expectations go.

One of my first incidents came when my daughter was three years old. This was going to be her first celebration of Halloween and I couldn't wait. I looked forward to taking her around our neighborhood for trick or treating. It was going to be the first time I'd been trick or treating since I was a kid and I was anxious to get my daughter started in the tradition. Since she was way too young to eat all that candy—yes, yes, I did allow her to eat candy (see Chapter 4 for more of my old despicable mothering)—I was relishing all the chocolate that would keep me happy through the first week of November.

Mostly though, this was going to be the first year she'd have a costume, and I had the perfect one picked out for her. It was a bee costume, but not just any bee costume. This was the very costume I wore when I played a bee in an ice skating performance when I was five. I had long lost the wings that went along with it, but I had dutifully saved the other pieces of this costume through various moves over the years. The black leotard base was a little discolored but not too badly, the top, made of yellow and black satin, looked as good as new, and the cute cap with the antennae on it still had all the sequins on it. My daughter had inherited her father's broad shoulders which meant this was the year the costume would fit her the best.

I allowed plenty of time on Halloween morning for her changing into the costume. She was happy to be a bee, although not super excited about it in the way I'd hoped. We were going to be spending the morning at a Halloween parade and a party at her pre-school. She'd get a chance to walk around the campus with her classmates and then return to their classroom for a cake and juice party. She'd be able to go home early, take a nap, and be ready to go trick or treating with me at the end of the day.

That was the expectation. Here is the reality. Although normally a very social girl, that day she was unusually quiet. She participated in the parade, but not with her usual enthusiasm. She didn't eat very much at the party either—yes, she rejected the cake!--and was very happy when I told her it was time to go home.

She fell asleep on the ride to our house and went right to her bed as soon as she walked in the door, again very usual behavior for her. She ended up sleeping straight through the night and by morning was back to her usual happy self.

I was disappointed that we didn't get to go around our neighborhood. It wasn't just the candy; I think I also wanted to show off this terrific little girl in her second generation bee costume and was sad I lost out on that opportunity. I found out years later that she was afraid of all those crazy costumes as she really didn't understand what was going on. Yes, that was a long time later—I was too clueless at the time to realize that might even be an issue.

This wasn't going to be the last time an expectation was to be dashed. What do you say when a seven-year-old girl rejects her father's gift of really expensive Guess jeans because she only wears dresses? Or when an eight-year-old boy rejects your favorite baseball team because he's decided he hates baseball? If you're wise, you run with it. You realize that ideal picture in your head must be revised. But that's okay because look at what's developed in its place: A young and fully forming human being with a mind of her/his own, a beautiful child who is totally whole, perfect and complete. Isn't that what you really wanted in the first place?

By Betsy Chasse and Debbie Spector Weisman

Chapter 17
The Single Mom

Debbie: Even if you're married, there are times you're going to feel like a single mom. Say your husband has a job that requires him to travel often or perhaps he's a real workaholic. You're going to find yourself at home alone, having to manage the house, the kids, and yourself at the same time. It's a big load.

It's natural that you're going to feel resentment. After all, he's out there doing his thing, free to go wherever he feels, and most importantly, he's spending his time in the company of *adults*. Meanwhile you're trying to figure out how you can console your daughter whose best friend just told her to get lost while your other two children are playing tug of war with the family cat. It's enough to drive you crazy.

Do yourself a favor. Please don't go crazy. Before you go off and say, "Oh that's easy for her to say," listen to this. I've been there. I've been that married single mom. When my kids were little my husband was busy building up a new company and that meant long nights and working on weekends. Often that meant going to school plays and piano recitals by myself.

Being a married single mom is not easy. But you can get through it. Here's how.

1. **Prevention.** No, I don't mean it as in not having kids in the first place. But some time between ditching the birth control and facing a brood of screaming brats, you're going to have to sit down with your husband and get a clear sense of your roles. Is he expecting you to do all the heavy lifting? If so, are you okay with that? This leads me to…

2. **Never make assumptions.** Too many married couples lose it because they simply assume that parenting is going to take care of itself. They don't stop to think of the *what ifs*. Actually that's not true. *You* probably do think about these things but your husband may just assume that you'll be around to pick up the kids from basketball practice or take them to the doctor appointments. That's fine if you're a stay-at-home mom who's

prepared to take on those assignments. But if you're working full time, like your husband, you'll need to decide *in advance* who's going to be responsible for the child rearing roles. And be happy about it.

3. **Ditch the resentment.** Take a deep breath and remember how you got here. You chose to get married. You chose to have kids. If you didn't do that advance planning and find yourself as the primary parent, then own it. You'll have to be the grown-up and find ways to cope. Remember that your husband does love you and the kids. He's just an incompetent nincompoop when it comes to raising them. Forgive him for this flaw in his character and move on. If you can't, then it's time to get a divorce and be a real single mom.

4. **Have a support system.** If your husband believes it's more important to play golf with his buddies than teach little Hannah how to throw a football, find someone who will. Maybe you can call on your brother, your father, your neighbor, or a friend

to help you with the things you can't do on your own. You don't have to do it alone.

5. **Get organized**. Let's say that your husband is a reasonably good parent to your kids. But he's often out of town on business trips and that means weekends home alone with the kids. Decide in advance on several activities you can do with them. Stress comes when there's no plan, and when there's no plan chaos is inevitable. If they're old enough, they can take part in the decision-making process, though I will admit you'll have to put your foot down and say no if all they want to do is go to Disneyland every weekend.

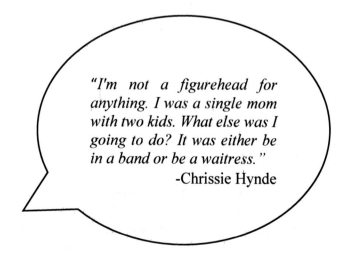

"I'm not a figurehead for anything. I was a single mom with two kids. What else was I going to do? It was either be in a band or be a waitress."
-Chrissie Hynde

By Betsy Chasse and Debbie Spector Weisman

Betsy: I am a single mom. I got divorced when my kids were six and three and a half, and for the first two years I was pretty much the sole everything, save for the every other weekend break. I had to work to support my kids and I had to work to raise them all on my own. There was no light at the end of the day, there was no daddy coming home eventually to give me a little time before bed or dinner. It was me, 24-7 and it was hard and scary.

When you first get divorced you have so many emotions already. For me the biggest wasn't the break up, it was the impact on my kids and the fear that I couldn't do it alone. There is a lot of guilt and shame at failing at marriage and the guilt and fear that you've failed your kids. UGH!

What did I do? I asked for help. I went to therapy, I asked my mom for help and I asked my friends. I knew that it takes a village to raise a kid (or two) (I mean Hillary said that didn't she?!) so I created a village and it paid off.

When you're a mom you already have a tendency to lose yourself in your kids; well, this gets magnified when you're a single mom. You don't make time for you and you constantly remind yourself, you don't have time, you've got to make up for the missing piece of your unit, you're playing dual roles and you often feel like you're missing some of the parts required to make this work. How can you keep the wheels moving if you're missing wheels?

For me, it started with seeing that, although my system was different and that maybe I didn't have it all, I could live like I did. Kids are pretty amazing and resilient and the old saying *happy Mommy makes happy kids* is very very true.

Early on in my divorce I received some advice that saved me. Your kids are used to one way of living and suddenly everything has shifted, and they are looking to you to see how to respond. If you flip out and panic, they will too. So don't panic. Talk to your kids about what's happening, what's going to change, what's not going to change, what you do know and what you don't know, and let them see you survive and thrive. When it doesn't work, let them see you laugh anyway.

It's also okay for them to see you struggle a bit, before you hit it out of the park. My kids watched me go from struggling to make ends meet, to thriving in my dream and you know what, it was the best thing I could have done for them. Five years after my divorce, my kids are proud of me. They learned that it's not always easy, but with a good attitude and hard work you can live your dream no matter your circumstances. They learned that heartbreak doesn't have to mean the end, it can also mean a new beginning.

The second and to me the most important piece of advice can be described as: Long term, short term. You cannot win every battle, but you can win the war, the war being the day you see your grown up kids are not so screwed up after all. It's totally okay that this Christmas isn't as big as when you were married, as long as it's fun. It's totally okay that you don't make it to every birthday party or event, as long as you engage your kids in learning to make decisions about what's important for the family.

Depending on their age (and it can work at almost any age) inviting your kids to participate in decisions--as long as they know you have the final word--empowers them. They feel like they didn't have a choice in the divorce, where they live, even when they see their dad, so any chance to allow them to feel part of the team helps. Giving them opportunities to make little choices for themselves, and god forbid, allowing them to be the wrong choices, is an amazing lesson for them. (Okay, seriously, I'm not saying allow your kids to leap off a cliff in order to test gravity for themselves.) But bringing them along when you're looking at a new place to live, or asking their opinion on how to re-decorate the house--especially their rooms--makes a big impact.

One last thing. For a long time I used the "I'm a single mom" card, a lot. I repeated that mantra over and over again, as if it gave me permission to fail, to be unhappy, to say "I can't, I'm a single mom." I wore it like a badge of honor and a noose all at the same time. It gave me permission not to go to yoga, not to buy those new shoes, not to, not to, not to.

I was talking with a friend who finally said to me, "I am so sick of hearing that you're a single mom. You act as if you're the first woman to have to raise kids alone. Get over yourself."

That little tough love from an honest friend went a long way. Even as I write this chapter I cringe at the sentence. Yes, I am single, yes, I am a mom, but it doesn't define me. Yes, I have challenges, but they don't weigh me down, they inspire me. One tiny shift in perspective and I am doing it, surrounded by support and love.

Chapter 18
Milestones You'd Rather Not Have... But Probably Will Anyway

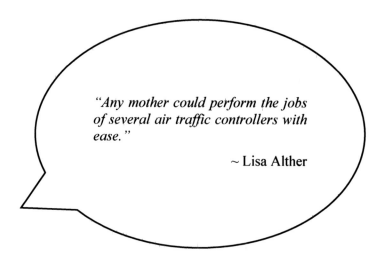

"*Any mother could perform the jobs of several air traffic controllers with ease.*"

~ Lisa Alther

We've already touched on the baby milestones that you can't help but track, those touchstones of growth like sitting up, rolling over, crawling, walking, and talking. As they get older there are other important childhood events that everyone cherishes such as the first day of school, the first Halloween, the loss of the first tooth, your child's first date.

By Betsy Chasse and Debbie Spector Weisman

Then there are the other "special" events, the kind that invariably happen even though you wish they wouldn't. Here's a short list to ponder.

1. **The first time you see real tears.** Of course your baby starts crying from minute one of life. It's the only way she knows how to communicate and you soon learn how to distinguish those sounds. At the beginning it's simple, either food, a clean diaper or a warm hug is wanted. Then one day you look up and it's not just a cry on your baby's face. There are tears, real wet ones dripping from those baby blues. The first time you see them it's a shock. Get ready. It won't be the last time you'll see them. There is nothing worse than seeing your child hurt and all we moms want to do is try and help them avoid the same pitfalls we fell prey to, but that my dear is futile. They are going to get hurt, they are going to feel the pain of loss, anger, sadness, confusion and sometimes instead of trying to fix it, sit with them and let them cry, let them feel and let them work

through it, their way, all the while standing at the ready with a box of Kleenex and a shoulder.

2. **Your first trip to the emergency room. Debbie:** Hopefully this is one you'll never have to experience. Nobody expects their child to be anything but perfect in any way. But accidents happen, illnesses flare up and suddenly you find yourself on the way to the emergency room. These things usually happen at night and invariably in winter when it's both cold and dark and you've been awakened from a pleasant dream of vacationing on a tropical island. Your child is screaming like an alley cat, your parental instincts are kicking in high gear and your mind naturally wanders to the worst case scenario. You're convinced that fever is the first stage of Ebola, that gash on the forehead is a precursor of the brain tumor you're sure is lurking on the other side of his skull. Your natural reaction is to panic, but this is the time to remember that you're a grown up now. You have a brain that can think rationally. Therefore, you bundle your kid up, remember to put clothes on yourself and

rush over to the emergency room where trained professionals can assure you that everything's going to be okay and that with a little Tylenol or a Band-Aid your child will be as good as new soon.

Betsy: When my daughter broke her arm I was riddled with guilt. You see she and I were on the monkey bars, and I was the one pushing her, standing underneath her ready to catch her. When I gave her a slight push she let go and well, I didn't catch her and down she went. I immediately saw her arm do things no child's arm should do. Everything went into slow motion and I went into a panic. (This does not help by the way).

After a few moments of both of us screaming, I got my shit together, gathered her into my arms, got my husband and headed for the ER. There she laid, actually calmer than I was when a nurse came in. Her dad was there, and to be honest, he's much better with hospitals than I am, so I left the room. Yep, I left her with the professionals because my stress and anxiety wasn't helping. The truth is, most of the time, your kid is going to be fine, and it's the moms who need the fainting chair. If you can, try to bring someone with you to enable you to step out in the hall and scream or cry. Otherwise, trust that everything will be okay and you'll have a good story for next year.

3. **The first time you hear "I hate you". Debbie:** That first day when you're holding your newborn you can't imagine anything but love pouring out of that little lump of flesh. Just remember that image. You're going to want to have that memory seared into your brain for the day when she looks at you with venom in her eyes and spits out the three most cutting words a parent can hear: I hate you. In that moment it's going to be hard to realize it, but deep down she really doesn't mean it. The next day you're likely to be awakened by a hug and a poignant "I'm sorry" that will melt your heart and enable you to remember why you had her in the first place.

4. **The first time something important gets ruined. Debbie:** We haven't talked much about baby proofing in this book. I

guess we just assume you're smart enough to know how to keep your home free of the obstacles that can cause harm to your child. There are also plenty of books out there that have lots of practical advice that we don't need to repeat here. But just because you've made your home as safe as a ball pit doesn't mean that nothing bad will ever happen. I'm talking about things like that sweet devil jumping up and down on your iPad, knocking over a glass of grape juice on your best linen tablecloth, flushing your favorite necklace down the toilet, or knocking your smartphone into the garbage disposal. There's just one way to deal with all of this. Repeat to yourself three times: Shit happens, shit happens, shit happens.

5. **The first time you're caught naked. Debbie:** Remember those pre-baby days when you romped around the house with little or nothing on and nobody cared? From the day the baby comes home you can kiss those days goodbye forever. (By the time the kid's grown up you probably won't want to scamper about sans clothing anymore.) You're extra careful to never

It Came Out of my Vagina! Now What?!

leave your bedroom in the morning without full coverage. Nevertheless, accidents do happen. Mine came the day I thought I could get away with taking a shower while my daughter was napping. I didn't feel the need to lock the bathroom door and you can imagine my surprise when I opened the shower curtain and saw that surprised little mouth say, "Hi, Mommy."

Betsy: I on the other hand have no issue being naked in front of my kids, still, I mean I show some restraint, but I also want my kids to not fall prey to the whole shame the body game our society plays. Since my son was a baby he has used the squeezing of my breast as a soother, as he got older this got a little weird, especially in public. I just kept moving his hand from my boob to my heart. Okay not as squishy (I mean what boy doesn't love a good squishy breast) and would say, "Those are Mommy's now and you need to respect my body."

I don't want him to be the creep at school and I want him to respect a woman's body. I don't want him to have some weird Oedipus complex when he's older and well, you know, wants to squeeze the breast of someone other than his mom. There are a lot of issues around bodies for both boys and girls. I hope I'm teaching them to love and respect theirs and others.

6. **The first time you're embarrassed in public.** This can happen in so many ways. **Debbie**: Mine came when we took our toddler son to his first grown up party. Everyone thought he was cute and adorable and the host was delighted to have him there—until he climbed onto his lap and puked all over his chest.

   Betsy: Here's the deal, your kid is going to do and say some really embarrassing stuff, get used to laughing at it, if the other adult can't figure out they're a kid, then screw them.

7. **The first unwanted pet. Debbie:** This could be the roly poly scooped up from the front lawn, the snail from the backyard. In my case it was a little lizard which we named Popcorn. We bought it a cage, went to the pet store every other day to buy it crickets to eat and otherwise just stared at it. Here's the thing

to know about all pets, whether it's the cute puppy you adopt from the shelter or the stray insect retrieved from the neighborhood: the care and feeding is going to be done by you. I drew the line when my daughter insisted on having two rats—which she named Thelma and Louise--in her bedroom. I out and out refused to have anything to do with them. To her credit she really did take care of them by herself until they mercifully died about a year later. I was so pleased with her maturity in this task that I gave in to her desire to preserve the little critters in the refrigerator because someday she wanted to dissect them. I didn't want to have anything to do with that scientific discovery either and after a few months neither did she and we were able to banish the rats from our lives forever.

8. **The first time they realize there's no tooth fairy. Debbie**: This is a tough one, as I honestly believe more kids buy into the tooth fairy than either Santa Claus or the Easter Bunny. Somehow their kid radar suspects those holiday icons are the clever makings of myth and marketing. But the tooth fairy is

different. Hard cold cash is involved and there's real magic when a tooth under the pillow transforms into dollars. When that day comes that they realize there's a human involved, it's time to turn it into a teachable moment. Life is hard. Life is tricky. You are easily fooled and it's time for you to wise up.

9. **The first bout with lice. Debbie**: I always thought that nit picking was one of those odd expressions without meaning until the day my daughter came home with lice embedded in her long hair. They're an equal opportunity pest and trying to remove those things from a screaming kid's head is torture for both of you. It doesn't matter if you've got the cleanest house on the block or if you force your kids to shower three times a day. No one is immune from a lice outbreak.

10. **The first F on a report card. Debbie**: Again, you expect your kid to be perfect in every way. But not every child is destined to be the next Bill Gates. One day when you least expect it, your little darling will come home with a pout on her face and

hand you a test paper with the 6th letter of the alphabet emblazoned at the top. To my mind this can be looked at like a weed. If you pull it up quickly and get all the roots, it'll never come back.

Betsy: I don't believe in grades, even if the public school system does. I have a rule, if you're doing your best and working hard I really don't care what someone else thinks. If one of my kids is struggling, I work with them, I get them a tutor, whatever they need. I don't get mad I get help.

11. **The first time you forget to pick up your kid. Debbie:** Yeah, yeah, I know you believe you're incredibly responsible and this would never happen to you. But…you are human and you're bound to screw up. Kiss them profusely when you reunite, swear up and down it will never happen again, and mitigate your guilt with a trip to the toy store.

Betsy: This happened to me, I was working and I didn't realize the kids got out of school early. I got a call from the school office (The horror! My perfect Mommy image ruined!) I beat myself up all the way to school, almost to the brink of tears until I walked into the office, which was full of about 25 kids in the same boat, all having a blast.

12. **The first F bomb. Debbie:** You will think you've gone to great lengths to keep your potty mouth closed until after your kid's asleep. But in today's information world you're not the only input for your child's inner computer. He's going to pick up words you'd rather he didn't know and you might never learn his source. In any event, this much is true. He'll find a way to launch that nasty word at the most inappropriate time.

    Betsy: I have an issue with "good" words and "bad" words, especially nowadays when bad means good and most words are reduced to one letter. I also have quite a potty mouth. Instead of trying to hide it, I taught my kids the proper use of a good "f" bomb. Hey there is a time and place, right? As of now, my kids haven't whipped it out in front of a priest (not that I have a priest), and oddly enough the allure of uttering such words is a whole lot less. It's still fun, but my kids are free to cuss at will, as long as it's used properly, like when they stub their toe or something. A good "FFFFF" is scientifically proven to make the pain go away.

13. **The first time there's trouble at school.** **Debbie:** Hopefully your child will be great at following the rules and in getting along with his classmates. Unfortunately, it doesn't always work that way and one day you'll get a call to come to school for a conference. I'll never forget the time my son was in sixth grade and my husband and I met with the principal and my son to discuss a fight he had with another boy. "This is your first strike," the principal told my son. He looked up at her with the most soulful look of contrition on his little freckled face. "Can't we just call it a foul ball?" he asked. We all laughed, of course. He still got detention.

Betsy: I have been told that when my brothers and sisters were young and in school, when one got in trouble they all did, boy did this cause quite a raucous in my house. Luckily they've let go of the medieval policy and I think teachers are better at dealing with kids and their issues. I'm an involved school parent, I volunteer, get to know the teachers and principle and this goes a long way when your kids act up, it's going to happen, for me I try and listen to my kids version as well, a few times it's come out that in fact they were wrongly accused and I got a lot of Mommy points from them and the teacher, but don't always assume your kid is innocent either, because it's absolutely possible that on that day, your kid was a butt.

14. **The first time you're "caught in the act"**. **Debbie:** Again, you think you'll go the extra mile in waiting to do the nasty until inquiring eyes are far far away. But one day when you least expect it, she'll wake up unexpectedly, and instead of it being your husband you hear, you'll by startled when it's a soft sweet voice that murmurs, "More. More. More."

Betsy: Seriously, lock the door!

Chapter 19

Other Mommies Weigh In: Opinions are like Vagina's every lady has one and we'd like to share some thoughts from other Mommies about their parenting experiences.

Top Ten Things They Don't Tell You About Giving Birth

By: Kevra Cherne

1. **You don't forget the pain.** Ever. Ever. Ever. Ever. That's just something they tell you to make you feel better. You will, however, forget the pain while having sex in the future and will likely end up pregnant again. There's that.

2. **Walking does really help labor, however, they don't tell you NOT to walk two miles in labor.** You might think that is "common sense" though YOU'RE IN LABOR so common sense really doesn't kick in here.

3. **When you walk two miles in labor, you show up at the hospital dilated to eight cm, which means:**
   No Drugs For You. Imagine the movie *Fast and Furious* …you're about to experience it with your vagina.

4. **Do not have your grandmother drive you to the hospital** (especially if she has a heavy foot on a regular day). Though you do get to practice your breathing.

5. **Your water may not break.** You are still in labor.

6. **Your body will want to push with or without you.** It feels better if you push. Medical professionals will not always want you to push and you will still want to do it anyway. I will let you figure this one out on your own.

7. **You don't effin' care if you have a candle burning or music playing.** Also, I wouldn't suggest anyone put any hands, etc.

near your mouth (even if it's to feed you ice chips) in hard labor as you will likely bite it off.

8. **You will not go home in your regular sized jeans.** Don't even bring them; your ego is not up for it. Trust me. I took it for the team on this one.

9. **After you push out your baby they will ask you if you want to hold and kiss her.** She is full of blood and goo. She is gross. I recommend a peck at most. Or have your partners wipe off the head quickly so you don't look like an ass. You don't care, you just pushed out a watermelon that will now keep you up for the next six months at least every night.

10. **When you're being stitched up with eighteen stitches because she came out too fast and they ask if you'd like to try breastfeeding, the proper response is, "Nothing else is touching me today! She will be bottle fed!"** And that is just fine.

By Betsy Chasse and Debbie Spector Weisman

Surviving Other Family Members
By Marla Keller

Kayla, our first-born, was a birth control pill baby. How does that happen? Apparently, our fertility knew no bounds. She made her surprising grand debut, on January 10, like the great Theater Arts graduate she became, a little bit earlier than expected. Like four weeks early. No complications, no fuss, and in and out of the hospital in eleven hours.

Jami I were in a bit of shock, and not really prepared, although my body must have known what was up because I made several casseroles like a crazy lady and put them in the freezer two days before her arrival. The kitchen looked like a tornado had passed through when I was finished. Her room was far from ready, and our families lived states away. We were left to fend for ourselves for a week. I was 21 years old, didn't have younger siblings, and I had never babysat more than once or twice in my life. Talk about the blind leading the blind. I was a child raising a child!

It Came Out of my Vagina! Now What?!

Looking back, that quiet time we had to spend together, just the three of us, was so blissful and beautiful. Even though this wasn't our plan—my mom and dad had blocked out two weeks to be with us around the birth, and Jami's mom had airline tickets purchased—I recommend this to all mothers expecting their first child. Bringing family in right away always complicates an already hormone-frenzied new mom!

But the second child, especially if they are sixteen months apart? That's a whole other animal.

> **Tip #1:** *Take at least 4 days to a week to get to know your new little family. Dads should always take at least this time off completely from work and other outside activities to allow for your precious little household to gel.*

By the time my parents arrived a week later, Jami and I had settled into a very comfortable routine with Kayla. Dad stayed for a week, and Mom for two. I was grateful for the help, and for the gentle tidbits of advice my mom offered. I feel grateful that she

By Betsy Chasse and Debbie Spector Weisman

intuitively knew that I was already pretty overwhelmed with a new little one, and she did not pile on control about how I needed to parent. Not yet, anyway...

When Jami's family visited for his graduation, his mom's approval of certain things most definitely revealed her disapproval of others, like the fact that I was allowing Kayla to have her pacifier for too long (Kayla was 5 months old and loved her "passy"), or that I was giving her the "wrong" baby foods to start out with because, you know, there was a right way to do it. After all, she was the expert having her own children, and was seven to ten years older than three of her siblings and also a childcare provider for many years.

It was also hard to swallow that she wouldn't tell me this, but would grab Jami and have quiet discussions in the other side of the room, letting him know her concerns. Ughhh! And guess who was on the receiving end of my physically and emotionally exhausted tirade against my mother-in-law? Jami. Poor Jami. It really pissed me off that he took *her* side! I just can't even.

It Came Out of my Vagina! Now What?!

Tip #2: *Have your partner's back no matter what! Even if you don't agree with your partner, at least have their back while engaging in conversation with your family, then have a private conversation with your spouse when the time is right.*

During the first sixteen months of Kayla's life we visited my family several times, and also flew out to Maryland to visit Jami's family once. I was the first of my siblings to have children, even though my brother and sister were older than me, and apparently *much* wiser, particularly as it related to raising children. Jami and I were constantly bombarded with how incompetent we were in this department. Mind you, I was on the cliff's edge of diving headlong into a serious case of OCD when it came to the perfection of my child, my home, my husband…you get the picture. I was a perfectionistic, "rather be right than in relationship" bitch. For the love.

When we stayed at my family's homes if Kayla so much as looked at the beautifully stacked magazines, or reached out to simply touch the leaves on one of the houseplants, I was pierced by a death-stare that said, "She better not even..." We had taught her from the first time she could pull herself up to stand next to the coffee table that she was not allowed to touch anything on the coffee table unless we put one of her toys there for her. Poor kid. She was so good. Really, she was an angel. She would look, touch gently, look at us to see if it was okay, and then proceed or not. Rarely she would dishevel the magazines, but never did she do any damage to them.

On one particular occasion Kayla was looking at a miniature adobe replica of San Javier Mission on the mantle next to my sibling's fireplace, and she reached out to touch the cross. Much to her distress--and mine--it fell off its precarious perch. My sister-in-law was distraught, glancing at me with the look of death, and in her haste to make sure the miniature was not harmed in the handling, Kayla was afraid and began to sob uncontrollably. I, of course, apologized profusely for the two seconds I had my eyes off of her, and ran over to do damage control, only to discover that the cross fit right back neatly into its place and was meant to be dismantled for storage and/or moving. Oy vey!

I spent too much time worrying about Kayla being perfect, and not enough time simply loving her and allowing her to explore her environment safely with appropriate guidance. I was so afraid of being disapproved of by my family, and friends, that I lost out on a lot of cuddle and love time, and our daughter lost out on the joy of discovery without the fear of getting in trouble.

To be fair, my siblings have apologized profusely for their unrealistic and harsh expectations regarding our parenting. This happened about ten years after they had their own children. Surprise! Having children is not for the faint of heart.

When we visited Jami's family in Maryland for Thanksgiving when Kayla was ten months old. I thought maybe this trip would be different, and that Jami would stand up for me and we would be our own little family unit. Not. So. Much. It seemed that everything I did as a mom wasn't good enough, or was downright wrong. There weren't a lot of words around this, just looks. I had tried so hard to gain their approval and love, and here I was failing again.

I didn't have the tools at the time to allow their actions to be theirs, and not own them as if I had done something wrong. I was the outsider, and they wanted to make sure I knew that. I don't believe they were being malicious; it was just that they had been so disappointed that I took Jami away from them that they couldn't forgive me for that.

It took a few years, but Jami discovered the importance of putting our little family above the needs of his parents, and what a relief that was.

> **Tip #3:** *Balance. Be aware of putting your family of origin's desires above the needs and emotional health of your kids (and your spouse). In the ideal hierarchy of life your spirit (self-care much?) needs to be in the top position, then your significant other, THEN THE KIDS, then your work, and then other family. When you put your family of origin and their demands on you above your spirit, spouse and children you lose out on the most important connections in your life.*

It Came Out of my Vagina! Now What?!

At sixteen months old, Kayla became a big sister. Jami and I joke that Ariel was our "condom baby" since the condom was left unopened on the nightstand. Oops! What an awesome "oops" it was. I was in labor for a whopping four hours, and she crowned so quickly that the nurse was panicking and couldn't get a hold of my doctor. Being the good co-dependent that I was I didn't push, even though, dear God, I was desperate to! I waited for my doctor to walk in the room before I pushed, and within three contractions she was out, purple, not breathing. Scariest thing in my life. When I finally heard her cry it was the sweetest sound ever.

My mom and dad were already visiting us, since Ariel was 2 days late (l o n g e s t two days of my life, by the way!) My mom and dad took turns watching Kayla while I was in labor, until the actual birth, and then my mom and Jami were in the delivery room while my dad was with Kayla.

Dad was pretty anxious and very adamantly stated over and over again that he wasn't good with kids under the age of eight. He was actually better than he thought with them, but was fairly inpatient with them as well as being critical of our parenting skills.

By Betsy Chasse and Debbie Spector Weisman

My parents stayed with us for four days until my mother-in-law flew in to help us out. I was drained physically and emotionally distraught when my mom and dad drove away. I sat on the porch with my jammies and hormonal wreckage sobbing my little heart out. I almost could not bear the thought of heading inside the house to the cold stone feel of my mother-in-law. It was icy. She was an incredible help though, and honored my desire to have Ariel wait four hours between feedings that Kayla had warmed to so quickly. I was so rigid that I couldn't recognize that Ariel was a different being from Kayla, and that she had different needs.

It was during this visit that Jami's mom told me, continually, that Kayla didn't need her pacifier any longer, and that it was time for me to take it away from her. I kept repeating that Kayla had experienced enough changes in her little life simply by having a new little sister that I was going to let her have her "passy" as long as she wanted it. I heard all about the possible damage to her teeth and that her reliance on it would never be outgrown so now was the perfect time to take it away. I decided to ignore her. I'm glad I did, although I have to admit I'm not sure if it was good parenting or stubbornness. I am a redhead and an Aries, and there can be fire and horns when I feel backed into the corner!

I wish I had the tools then that I have now. If I could have forgiven the older irritations and pain, my experience with my mother-in-law would have been better even if she hadn't changed a thing.

Tip #4: *Forgive your family for the hurts they have delivered on you. After working with thousands of people in the area of forgiveness, Jami and I have noticed a powerful and distinct pattern. Hurt and pain from the past that is held in our hearts actually prevents peace, personal power, and joy. Choosing to forgive allows us to see what we really want. This forgiveness is designed for you to be free. It's not for the person who hurt you, and it doesn't give them a free pass to continue to hurt you. It also doesn't let them get away with anything. You forgive for you and your heart to open up the space and the intention*

By Betsy Chasse and Debbie Spector Weisman

for better relationships over all. It's not easy, but it's worth it!

As the girls were growing older, I made a decision to grow emotionally, and began to heal from my own childhood pain and trauma. This allowed me to be less and less obsessed with perfection and approval, and to start having better boundaries with our families. The last summer we flew the girls back to Maryland to visit Jami's family was when Kayla and Ariel were in 5th and 6th grades. When the girls secretly called us crying because Grandpa wouldn't allow them to use the phone without asking, he wouldn't let them lock their door for privacy, and told us that he had raged at them several times that was the end of our visiting Maryland. For our family's emotional safety, Jami put his foot down and let his father know that, unless things changed and our boundaries were kept, we wouldn't be visiting.

When the girls were in Junior High we gave them the freedom to make decisions about their bodies and lives as co-decision makers with us. Naturally our families had a hay-day! They thought we had lost our minds to give our girls so many freedoms. They were mortified when we allowed—God forbid—Ariel to get her ears pierced. Then, everyone was traumatized that we allowed our girls to get tattoos at sixteen. The coup de gras was when we started allowing them to drink moderately with us so that they could learn how to handle alcohol *before* they went away to college. Holy cow, people! What kind of sacred cows were behind that judgment and criticism? Time for some tipping…

The more we chose to become our own people, and allow our girls to be their own people, the better boundaries we began to put in to place for our families of origin.

Tip #5: *Boundaries are tough, especially when you haven't taken the time to forgive. Following forgiveness, boundaries come easier and with no strings attached. Forgiveness leads you to the truth seen through the eyes of compassion, and truth leads you to better boundaries. Here are some great boundary-filled statements to remember:*

By Betsy Chasse and Debbie Spector Weisman

- *This is not okay with me.*
- *Help me understand.*
- *When you do this, I feel (three real feelings, not a story)…*
- *I need to think about this. Give me an hour and I'll get back with you with my decision.*
- *What did you mean by that?*

Whatever your situation is with your families of origin, you can utilize the tips above of support, balance, forgiveness, and boundaries and create a beautiful environment of love, peace, empowerment and joy all around you. Conflicts with family do not have to translate into despair, anger or confusion. When you are able to choose release, you will receive so much more in return.

Apparently, we didn't mess up our girls too badly. Kayla is a Theater Arts Boise State University graduate, living with the love of her life, and said just last week that she's happier than she's ever been. She exudes confidence and poise. Ariel has been married for three years to Preston, an amazing guy (he and Jami are besties and have a bromance going on there…) She has a great job at Idaho Power, and she is the embodiment of what we've been teaching her whole life allowing her intuitive old soul create connection and joy everywhere she goes. We are so proud; can you tell?

By Betsy Chasse and Debbie Spector Weisman

How My Son Learned to Use His Words
By Kate Gardner

He came out of my vagina on the 24th of February at around two o'clock in the morning after only a four-hour labor. I swear when that kid came out and looked up at me for the first time he was thinking, *Hi Mom. Get ready for an insane ride for the rest of your life.*

When they say a child is the best thing and worse thing that could ever happen to you they are not kidding! Let me shake the hand of the honest person who said that!

Suddenly the life you had of only having to think for yourself goes up in a puff of smoke and now you have a little person to place before everything else. Or in my case two, because my son Jordan was my second baby, and I assumed he would be as easy as the first one. Oh fuck me how wrong was I! You see two babies are never the same, and I was about to find that out big time.

My son is now all grown up, but the first sixteen years of his life was a love/hate reality that I had created for myself, and it nearly drove me insane. You see I always wanted to create a relationship with both my children where they could be open to express how they felt or what they wanted to say anytime they liked. I also wanted my children to develop great communication skills and quickly learn to speak properly so that by the time they were three years old and started attending nursery school people would be able to completely understand them. Rather than talk to them in a silly baby voice I wanted to give them the respect they deserved as little human beings and help their talking skills to enhance quicker.

Well, you know the term "unintended consequences"? Oh boy did I learn the consequences of letting that happen!

When he was around three and half years old, I was feeling generous and decided to take him out for lunch to treat him for being a good boy and not pulling his sister's hair for at least 24 hours. We were in a crowded café eating our lunch and quite a curvy lady sat across from us on the opposite table. Jordan swung his head round to her right like his head was attached to a spring and swung it full back at lightning speed right back to me again and said at the loudest decibel his voice could reach: "MUM! That lady over there is well fat isn't she?"

Oh my dear god! If there was ever a time I could grab a shovel and dig a hole in the center of the café and jump into to hide from the shame it was then. I could feel the entire café staring right at me, and all of them had gone totally deadly silent. I picked up my coat and the devil child and walked out with my cheeks burning brighter red than a baboon's ass.

Yes, I was annoyed and ashamed. I think what shocked me the most though was where the heck he learned the idea that somebody was fat? Had he picked up something that I had said about my own body at home? I know I had always talked to my kids like proper human beings, but was this my doing? Or was it something that was normal conversation among the three year olds at his nursery school?

As much as I wanted him to hold back on his major honest statements in public I had to realize that he was just doing what I wanted him to do all along--express his thoughts and feelings. Day in and day out I had told Jordan that he could tell me anything he

It Came Out of my Vagina! Now What?!

wanted, and I would never be cross as long as he was completely honest with me. Realizing it was me that had trained his brain to be so honest, I had to retrain my brain to recognize when this kid was about to put me in another potentially embarrassing predicament.

It didn't take me long before I soon became a master at it. I even stopped him once at the supermarket checkout before he could tell the whole supermarket how the cashier's boobs were so big they were nearly popping out her top. I had developed that mom radar to know what he was thinking and what he was about to say before he said it.

Most of the time, that is. When he did make these really honest statements in public I would place my hand lightly over his over his mouth to muffle the words from other people's ears. People must have thought that I was a nutter or totally understand what it was like to have a child in my life who was brutally honest.

Not only was Jordan honest; you couldn't shut him up for five minutes. If he couldn't speak all the time or hear his own voice he was not content. Even while traveling in the car his dad and I had to resort to using bribes to quiet him down. Yes! I admit that I am guilty of trying to bribe him to keep him quiet in order for my brain to process the 50 other things I should have been doing that day. We would say, "Jordan we will pay you to be silent for five minutes". He couldn't for the life in him be silent, and it was game over in less than two minutes because he would just start talking nonstop again.

This talking 600 words a minute habit didn't calm down anytime soon and it even drove us to the point where we totally refused to take him to the cinema. You see Jordan and his sister travelled to America a lot during their childhood and had the opportunity to watch a whole bunch of movies that had not yet been released yet in the U.K. Jordan with his "I can never stop talking habit" would completely relate the entire plot of the movie and even tell you—and everyone in the cinema who were in hearing distance of his voice--the best bits before they happened.

Even though all this constant talking and loud honest public statements were sometimes annoying I knew in my heart I wanted him to express what he thought and felt. Too many children on this planet are told to stand up and talk for the first two years of their lives, and then told to shut up and sit down for the rest of their lives which leaves them feeling like they are not allowed a voice or an identity.

Every child has an individual personality and will grow up into a completely different person from you. Yes, they will have similar interests to you and may like doing the same thing as you from time to time, but they are not you. Which is why these little individuals need to express themselves in what they do. We as the parents can guide them, protect them from harm and be there when they truly need us. However, it is not our job to control them and make them be a certain way or do a certain thing because it pleases us and not them.

We cannot squeeze children into boxes of the people who we want them to be. This results in placing a lot of pressure upon a little person and can leave a mark on them as they grow up and make them feel like a failure if they don't live up to the extremely high standards that are expected of them.

By Betsy Chasse and Debbie Spector Weisman

I know parenting is far from easy because I spent eleven years of my life bringing up two children by myself and running a business from home. There were days that I felt massive pressure. The questions would mount up. Can I really do this? Am I doing a good job? Parenting is a hard enough journey without thinking what we are doing is not good enough.

Life would be so much easier if every baby was born with a "How to bring me up" manual stuck to their chest when they popped into the world, but this is not how it happens. We have to figure this shit out for ourselves and do the best we can with the knowledge we have.

Listening to other stories from other parents can make you feel uncomfortable and scare you if you are about to become a parent yourself, and you could listen to them stories plus line up 100 parenting experts up outside your front door interview every one of them and you would still have a completely different experience from what all of them told you. Your parenting experience will not be the same as the person next to you, or your neighbor down the street, because the little human that you are parenting is unique and will bring his or her own unique personality to your family table.

Even though Jordan drove me insane with his honest and loud bold statements when he was younger I still allowed him to be so open and honest about what he thought. By allowing him to have freedom to bring that uniqueness to the world rather than bottle up it stopped his emotions exploding like a reactor and I didn't experience tantrums from him.

Looking back over his life now and asking myself could I have dealt with the situation in the café any better? Maybe, maybe not, who cares? There is no judge, jury, and executioner if you screw up, but if you do screw up (which we all do nobody is perfect) then be honest about it and be honest with yourself and admit that you could have handled it better, and at least that way you can move on and not carry the guilt through the rest of your years with you.

What I do know is that both my children grew up to be awesome young adults who felt they could live and speak the truth, and I learnt a whole bunch of things about myself along the journey with them.

By Betsy Chasse and Debbie Spector Weisman

I am now entering the next stage of having children in my life all over again because I recently became a grandma. My granddaughter Rosie came into the world in September this year, and it completely blew me away how much love you could have for your child's baby. I think it took me a whole week to get over the shock that my daughter now had a daughter of her own.

Will this new journey of grand parenting be completely different from the one I took with my own children? Of course it will! Rosie is not my child. I am now the grandparent and know what a massive impact grandparents can have upon a child's life. I feel as long as I am an inspiration to her like my grandparents were to me, then I know this little girl in three years' time will have a wonderful role model to look up too and to take whatever I teach her into her adulthood to benefit her and those around her and if I have anything to do with it they won't be a repeat café performance with her.

Food Inglorious Food
By Angela Mosely

I have food issues. Not serious, heart breaking food issues that require support and medical attention, but food issues that make me cry.

I've never been able to swallow mashed potatoes. Can't do it. Makes me gag every single time. Shredded coconut reminds me of fingernails. Can't eat it. I enjoy raw spinach, but cooked spinach makes me cry. I can't eat guacamole because it reminds me of....well, you don't want to know.

I guess it shouldn't have surprised or frustrated me when all three of our children showed similar food sensitivities. Our middle child, though, takes the matter to a level of food aversion perfection that can only be rivaled by my own absolute refusal to eat liver.

When we started Thing 2 on solid food, I had high hopes. His brother (Thing 1) happily ate the organic homemade mashed beets, carrots, beans, peaches, and bananas that I painstakingly prepared

By Betsy Chasse and Debbie Spector Weisman

in my very expensive super blender. Thing 1 would try everything and ate a wide variety of foods. Thing 2, on the other hand, steadfastly refused to consume any solid food except for oatmeal smothered in a precise blend of cinnamon and sugar (more sugar than cinnamon) and yogurt (but without any chunks of fruit). Oatmeal and yogurt for breakfast. Oatmeal and yogurt for lunch. Oatmeal and yogurt for dinner. Unless I mixed the oatmeal and yogurt. Then, he steadfastly refused to eat anything.

Playing the "here's the airplane spoon flying into your mouth" game didn't work. He clenched his jaws tightly shut.

Dressing up the fruits and veggies into little characters or fun patterns didn't work. He rearranged the patterns and played with the characters.

Bribing didn't work. "I not hungry, Momma," he would tell me when faced with the prospect of having to eat his dinner in order to get a cookie. What's left when the power of the bribe is gone?

I was desperate. I was distraught. I emailed our pediatrician, asking for her advice, though secretly I was afraid it could result in my mommy card being revoked. I went to the experts on

It Came Out of my Vagina! Now What?!

Pinterest, but I think Thing 2 was born with an advanced bullshit radar. It's as if he could (and still can) smell vegetables mixed into sauces or meatballs. He could sense fruit mixed into breads or muffins. He wouldn't touch any of it. I wasted too much time and money trying to make foods my kid would eat.

You might think I'm exaggerating the situation for the sake of great reading—but let me share the story of his first birthday to help you understand the mental anguish his eating habits and my mommy failure caused me. First birthdays are kind of a big deal, right? Many of us make the small cake (a smash cake, as they are sometimes called) for the little birthday babe. I happily made a small smash cake for Thing 2, and I was so excited to take pictures and video of him eating and playing with his first cake. After he finished his dinner (of oatmeal and yogurt—don't judge), I proudly placed the cake on the tray of his little booster seat, and Poppa grabbed the camera to start filming. Thing 2 looked at the cake. He looked at me as if to say, "Did you hide fruit inside that?"

Thinking that maybe he wasn't sure what to do, I took a bit of frosting on my finger and placed it on his lips. He made a face at me. Undeterred, I took a small bit of cake and icing on the tip of a fork and placed the bite in his mouth. I waited for his smile and excitement as he realized I had just placed this sugary confection in front of him and he didn't have to share it with anyone. I didn't have to wait long...but I didn't get a smile. He gagged and threw up. He choked. He spit. I nearly cried. My child threw up his first birthday cake (and his birthday dinner). What kid refuses birthday cake?!? My kid, apparently.

I gave up.

Then one day, acting on a hunch that maybe he had issues with texture (as I do), I gave him a smoothie. Sweet Clouds of Glory!! He drank it and asked for more. Fruit—he was eating fruit! And of course, vegetables, because I'm tricky like that. (Insert diabolical mommy laughter here.) He would eat spinach if I blended the hell out of it and mixed it with strawberries and banana and yogurt and put it in a cup he couldn't see through so he wouldn't know it was green. As long as there were no chunks of fruit or random vegetable leaves and he couldn't see the color of the smoothie, he would drink it.

It Came Out of my Vagina! Now What?!

Once I even made a super nasty smoothie, with raw garlic, because I was sick and thought the garlic would help me feel better. It helped me throw up. I gave the smoothie to Thing 2, and he drank it all right there where he stood next to me in the kitchen. Freak.

We had turned a corner. My eighteen-month old would now eat three things: oatmeal, yogurt, and smoothies!

As I thought about my own food aversions and the awful nights at my childhood dinner table as I struggled to swallow slimy cooked spinach or fighting back tears as I chewed liver that tasted and smelled (to me) like blood, I found a place of compassion for this little person. Yes, I also found frustration. Oatmeal and yogurt is a terrible nutrition plan! I have always taken the time to buy and prepare healthy foods and here was this one year old (then two year old, then three year old, and now four year old) refusing to eat the food I put in front of him. But in a way, I knew that I understood where he was coming from.

That's when I had a mommy epiphany. This beautiful boy, so dearly loved, is not going to starve himself. It is not in the nature of a child to willingly starve himself when food is offered.

By Betsy Chasse and Debbie Spector Weisman

Eventually, the will of a little boy breaks, and his hunger wins. At least, that's what they say. At any rate, I realized that it is his responsibility to feed himself (once weaned from nursing or the bottle), and it is my responsibility to provide healthy food and model good eating habits. It is also my responsibility to make sure that eating does not become an emotional battlefield, thus setting up patterns for dysfunction in the future.

I had these two powerful realizations, and the war over food shifted. I no longer felt responsible for a "mommy failure" because my child is the kid who won't eat whatever is put in front of him. I felt such relief when I gave him back his responsibility and decided to work only on mine. I set about trying to find ways to bring the joy back to our mealtimes, or at least diffuse the fights before they began. I found a few tricks that worked for us that didn't feel like bribing and seemed to make sense to Thing 2's highly developed sense of justice.

It Came Out of my Vagina! Now What?!

1. **The Age is the Bites**

   I developed a system in which every child at the table had to eat as many bites of each thing on their plate as they were old. Thing 2 was about three years old when I figured this one out. He had to eat three bites of meat, three bites of vegetables, three bites of fruit, etc. I did not specify how big a bite was, so my son still felt empowered to decide how much of something to put into his mouth. He would frequently hunt for the absolute smallest pieces of vegetable he could find—like one shred of a broccoli tuft, or a broken piece of half a green bean. But, the battles diminished because it made sense to him that if he was three, he had to eat three bites.

2. **The Dinner Winner Plate**

   If you have never seen this plate manufactured by Fred & Friends, please go find it as soon as possible. It's brilliant. I would alternate the food in each section, starting with the main protein in the "Start" position and then putting the vegetable in the second spot, the fruit in the third spot, then the protein, vegetable, fruit again, alternating up to the "Finish!" spot. It helped my son to still feel in control of his eating, while also forcing him to eat a variety of foods. (Because it's a game, though, it doesn't feel forced—it's genius!)

3. The Dessert First

Calm down. If dessert is one Hershey's kiss, or a small homemade cookie, is it really a crisis if the child eats dessert first or in the middle of the meal? By letting my son eat dessert before he finished his meal, I took away the leverage point and ended any fights before they began. He got to eat the sweet thing first, which often inspired him to eat three bites of everything else on his plate. It worked, and my kid has no lasting health problems from eating dessert first. I'm cool with it.

4. The Midnight Bailout

"But, Momma," he would frequently say as he refused to eat his dinner, "what if I wake up hungry in the middle of the night?" I would calmly reply, "That would be a bummer for you, wouldn't it? But it's my job to take care of you, so if you wake up, I will get you food." I know many parents disagree with me on this one. But if my child wakes for any other reason in the middle of the night, I go to them and attend to their need. Hunger is no different. Mind you, I don't make a meal at 2:30 in the morning. Nighttime waking's for hunger get met with a piece of bread and some water. It's not my son's favorite thing to eat, but he will tolerate it. I think what he is looking for when he asks this question is the reassurance that I will not let him starve. I am bigger than he is, in authority over him, and he wants to know that I will take care of him. Often, when we have this little conversation he responds with relief and doesn't wake up hungry in the middle of the night.

5. **The Lunch for Breakfast**

I love eating breakfast for dinner. When I was growing up, it felt like a rebel thing to do: eating the "wrong" meal for dinner. Just recently, though, I have started giving Thing 2 the foods he asks for. Frequently, he requests a cheese sandwich for breakfast, along with a glass of milk. That's a perfectly fine meal, and it has lots of protein. But my mind thinks that it's a meal for lunch, not breakfast. Nevertheless, I'm trying to suspend my definition of *appropriate meals* in order to make sure that my son eats. I'm trying to think more in terms of *appropriate foods*, eaten at regular intervals throughout the day. I'm pretty sure that's a principle most diets teach, so I think I'm on the right track.

6. The Ebb and Flow Pattern

My children do not eat consistently, especially Thing 2. Perhaps you've noticed this about your kids, too. One day, Thing 2 is starving all day long, and I can't get food in his hands fast enough. The next day, he eats yogurt and half a piece of bread. That's it—all day. I decided to stop fighting whatever this weird feast or famine pattern is. I try to feed him at consistent times, but I'm no longer tied to the clock. If he ate lunch around noon and wants dinner at four, sometimes I'll give it to him. I would rather have him eat early than have a face-melting, crabby mess at 6 pm because his blood sugar is too low and I've been ignoring his pleas for food in favor of following my schedule. (Trust me, Thing 2 takes face-melting crabbiness to new levels of grandeur. I'm not a fan of it. I prefer to diffuse that nuclear bomb before it goes off.)

It seems that feeding our children is a process that is fraught with loads of mommy guilt. Breastfeeding is better than bottle-feeding. Organic homemade food is better than McDonald's takeout. The whole family gathering around the table to dine and converse peacefully together is better than feeding people when they are hungry. As I've fumbled my way through these eating struggles, I've come to realize that Thing 2 may have more awareness of what his body requires than I do. Sometimes, that's hard for us mommas to say, "My child knows himself better than I do." But it is true.

It is also true, I think, that part of my job is to teach my children how to take responsibility for keeping their bodies healthy and well-fed. Trying to strike the balance between recognizing my child's own awareness and fulfilling my parenting responsibility is a delicate dance. I try to do it by presenting healthy choices and fun choices, too, because eating can be fun—and I leave the eating up to him.

By Betsy Chasse and Debbie Spector Weisman

Although he would still eat yogurt at every meal if I offered it (as long as there are no chunks of fruit in it), Thing 2 no longer likes oatmeal. Finally, he'll eat meat and single tufts of broccoli crowns, and barbeque sauce. Lots of barbeque sauce. We're making progress, my friends. I'm hopeful that when he's ready, he will explore new textures and flavors, and he'll end up realizing how many wonderful foods there are to eat. On that day, it will be his choice, and he'll embrace it completely. Until then, I will not stress myself out over his eating drama.

You shouldn't stress yourself out about your kid's eating, either. Make good choices in the foods you offer, and let them make choices about what to eat. You got this, Momma.

Repeat after me, "I will not stress myself out….I will not stress myself out…I will not stress myself out…"

Sex After Baby
By Tanya Lynn

After hearing horror stories from practically every woman I knew about how painful sex was after giving birth, I felt apprehensive.

"Make sure you lube up."

"You're going to be dry."

"I had a C-section and it still hurt!"

I did what any woman who was planning for the worst would do: I called Kimberly for a pelvic floor massage to get me ready.

Yes, you read that right. I called a woman to give the inner walls and lips of my vagina a good rub down and stretch out before the big game.

"There is no way I'm letting some woman enter you before me!" Brent, my husband, said to me when I told him that morning about my appointment later that day.

"But it's going to hurt. I need to prepare, babe," I replied.

By Betsy Chasse and Debbie Spector Weisman

"No way. We're doing this right now before she comes over," he said, taking my hand and leading me to our bedroom.

Sex for us has, for the most part, been like a cat and mouse game, where we take turns being the hunter and the prey.

We were together for only three months before I got knocked up. Imagine for moment having really amazing sex for only 90 days and then everything changing drastically.

For the first trimester, the idea of sex nauseated me. He smelled weird.

I felt like I wanted to throw up on him. I just wanted to sleep.

I can't remember sex during the second trimester. It was sporadic during the third.

I was as eager to get the party started again as he was. I wanted to feel that connection. I had almost forgotten what it was like for us to connect like that. My biggest fear was that we had lost it and we would be one of those couples that became live in roommates instead of lovers. That there would be no time or I would be too tired.

It Came Out of my Vagina! Now What?!

With a grin, I dragged my feet, "No … come on, babe! Let's wait till after!" I followed him anyway.

"Please grab the lube!" I instructed.

"What for?"

"Because it's going to hurt!"

"We don't need any lube."

"Yes, we do! I'm not doing this unless you get it!"

"Okay fine."

"Ehhhhhhh. I don't want to do this!"

"It will be fine."

"Kiss me dammit!"

"Okay."

"Wait! Ouch! That hurts!"

"I'm not even touching you!"

"Ehhhhhh. This is too much for me!"

By Betsy Chasse and Debbie Spector Weisman

"Just relax …"

"Don't tell me to relax! I had a nine pound baby come out of this vagina!"

"Well then this should be nothing."

"Babe, this is so traumatic right now! Oh my god oh my god!"

"I'm in."

"You're in?"

"Yes, I'm in."

"Ouch!"

"How can you say ouch when you didn't even know I was in?"

"Because now it hurts! Stop!"

"Okay I'm stopping."

He's lying on top of me. I'm breathing hard. I try to soften and relax my pelvic floor.

"Okay, easy please."

It Came Out of my Vagina! Now What?!

"Oh babe, it feels so good to be back inside of you. Oh babe. Mmmmmmm. It's all tight and warm. Mmmmmm."

"Really? It's tight? I thought it was going to be all stretched out?"

"No, I think she's better than before. Mmmmm, babe."

I laughed. This wasn't so bad after all. The lube helped. As long as he didn't press on the scar tissue, we were all good.

Later that day, Kimberly came over. Now to give you a little background, Kimberly is a professional pelvic floor masseur who came highly recommended by three women. I hired her a day before I went into labor to work out all the tension in my vagina. I screamed, cried and howled with pain as she worked.

I was desperate to get that baby out of my body at that point, and I tried everything to do it from the vaginal massage, castor oil, sex and rubbing my nipples.

Then Brent suggested his method. "Come on babe, let's have sex. It will induce labor."

"Babe, really? But you're so … big. I don't want to smash the baby."

"You won't. Let's try a new position."

"But babe …"

"We're doing it. Let's go."

We tried reverse cowgirl that day and he loved it. I mean, really loved it.

"You don't even look pregnant. And your ass. My god. Why didn't we find this position before?"

After Kali was born and once we got over the initial test run and Kimberly opened me up, I was ready to start easing back in and exploring.

The next time Brent made his advance, I met him in full stride. Except this time, Kali tuned into mama like a psychic. She knew exactly what we were up to—and she wasn't having it.

It Came Out of my Vagina! Now What?!

As soon as we were humping away, she started crying. Hard. Now this is a baby who rarely cried. Yes, we have an angel baby. But call her jealous, she was not about to let mama get knocked up again and ruin her parade. She needed all the loving she could get from me, and she was going to make sure no little brother or sister was coming any time soon.

As soon as I picked her up, she stopped. Just like that. *Mama, you are NOT having another one of my kind. Not over my dead body.*

"If we are going to do this, we've got to put her in the other room. This is terrible, having her in the same room as us doing it!"

"But she was asleep. Just put some pillows in front of the bassinet so she can't see us."

"No, we're putting her in her crib. And we can do it when we know she's *definitely* asleep."

Spontaneous sex? Not anymore.

Now when I put the baby down for a nap, even though I'm exhausted and wanting my own nap, I've got to muster up the energy for a quickie, throwing a Hail Mary to go for the touchdown before she catches us thumping away.

It's like high school all over again, sneaking your boyfriend over and hoping not to get caught by your parents, except this time, you are the parent.

As my mom would say, "Payback."

If you just got the shudders thinking about this, don't worry. I'm at the eight-month mark and we've found our groove. We are able to find the time for pleasure. We have date nights. We've even have had one night alone when Kali had a sleepover at my parents' with her older cousin.

Things are so juicy again that we're ready for #2. This time, I know that even if we take another hiatus during the next pregnancy, we'll find our groove with one another once again. All it takes is some time, patience, and a whole lot of lube.

It Came Out of my Vagina! Now What?!

Happy Mom Happy Baby, Confident Mommy, Calm Child
By Kim Somers Egelsee

I remember when I was pregnant with my first daughter Noella, (I have two daughters now; Nia and Noella), I thought I would keep up my current pace of working, my wild social life, (extensive bar hopping, rock concert going and all), fitness, traveling, side hobbies, career, projects, and travel. I had a college degree in speech communication and a teaching credential as an education specialist, and I was working as a special education teacher at a middle school full time. I also had the side project and passion of being in an entertainment rock group that also modeled and hosted events with a focus on educating the public about going vegetarian and adopting an eco-friendly lifestyle and I was even life coaching a bit on the side to help and be of service to others.

On my way to work as a special education teacher, I would pass by a local preschool and plan the future of dropping the baby off five days a week, eight hours per day, thinking it would be no problem. I imagined how I would easily and effortlessly glide through motherhood with style, grace and a positive attitude. I would picture myself going on weekly date nights with my husband looking fabulous, feeling stress free with my calm, giggly, happy new baby.

After a pretty difficult pregnancy with very bad asthma symptoms, quite a bit of weight gain, and severe sciatica, my beautiful chubby baby girl with a dimple in her chin and dark hair was here via C-section (due to her being breech; which means upside down). I did have this intense powerful love for Noella that was indescribable from the get go of being pregnant, and even more so the minute I saw her eyes.

However, I could barely walk, let alone bar hop or go to concerts. I was thrilled to finally be a real mommy, but overwhelmed with all of the tasks, care and responsibility suddenly thrown onto me. I began feeling anxious and hormonal at even the smallest of events such as taking my new little friend with me to the car wash, doctor or the store. I was overweight, bloated, my skin had broken out like a teenager from the hormones, and nothing looked good on me, let alone like I had style.

I was also having a horrible time with breast feeding. I was feeling not good enough, lost and let down. I wasn't sure how to handle this, so I did what many of us moms do. I called in the expert; my own mom, with whom I am extremely close. She started coming over a few times a week, as did my Mother-in-law, to help me, teach me, direct me and get me back to somewhat of a life balance, self-care, happy and confident new mommy mode.

I began to truly see the evidence that a happy mommy is a happy baby, and a confident mom equals a calm child. I still had five months before going back to work, which allowed me time to read parenting books, articles in magazines and on the internet, and asking my mom friends (and luckily my husband's brother and best friend are both doctors) all for advice. Additionally, yes the instincts kicked in on what to do and how to do it. I started to take a little bit of time for myself when I could to practice self-care with a nap, a massage, a bubble bath, have a glass of red wine, read, and actually exercise. I enrolled in a moms and babies yoga class. The

By Betsy Chasse and Debbie Spector Weisman

weight began coming off, my face cleared up, clothes started to fit better, and I felt more and more like me. My awesome husband and I also made sure to go on date nights, which ensured the passion stayed in our marriage as well.

Noella started to get out of the newborn "crying" phase, began to smile, laugh and move around more and more. This gave me real evidence that a happy mom means a happy baby.

I became very attached to my new little girlfriend, who looked at me adoringly with her big toothless smile and the dimple in her chin. I loved being with her, even with the lack of sleep from her waking up every two hours nightly. (Yes, she did this until almost age two, and I breast fed her just about that long!) I knew I would soon have to return to my work as a special education teacher for moderate to severe disabilities; which meant many children in wheelchairs with a lot of heavy lifting, fifty hours plus per week very soon. I was also required to do the second section of my education specialist credential, (a focus on educational psychology), which would require about eighteen more months of college. I felt uneasy.

It Came Out of my Vagina! Now What?!

Although I liked my job, and loved the kids that I worked with, no longer did the prior idea of day care daily for my baby inspire me. In fact, I felt freaked out by the idea of her being away from me at all. Additionally, I had always felt a whisper of something else being my life purpose. I did not yet know what that was. I was very happy, but there was something else out there that I was called and meant to be doing. I wanted to be home with my angel, or at least in a job working from home. This was not an option for my husband, who owns a very busy law firm, which actually specializes in special education law.

The day finally came when Noella turned five months old, and I had to return to work. I was a complete mess. I literally was crying, throwing up and feeling extreme anxiety all at the same time. I almost felt like I had to go to the hospital. My husband comforted me, reminding me that Noella wouldn't even be with a babysitter, or at a day care, but instead would have quality bonding family time with my mom or mother-in-law on the days I worked. However, since I only wanted her with family members, and didn't know of any babysitters, this was a huge challenge that required five hours of driving per day. Each day I would drive one hour to my moms or mother-in-law, one hour back to work, one hour back to pick up baby, and then two hours in traffic back home.

The five hours per day was intense, insane and almost unbearable. I began calling in sick at least once per week from the pressure. My hormones, mom emotions and love for her were overtaking and overwhelming me. I managed to get to work, and get through the day, pumping breast milk with a hand held pump that made me feel like a cow giving milk in the tiny staff bathroom, focusing on doing my job well, but also counting the minutes until I could hold her again.

As the weeks passed, I got into a routine. The anxiety and sadness drifted away (thank goodness), and I began to focus on doing an excellent job as the special education teacher that I was, but was still very tired and stressed out from all of the driving.

Besides my main full time job as a teacher, I mentioned I was following passions of side projects in entertainment and in life coaching. I started to realize that if I truly wanted life balance, and quality time with my family, as well as time to focus on my truest passions and possibly find a new purpose, I had to let this job as a special education teacher go. My required year was almost up. The crazy driving was almost over. With the persuasion of my Dad and my husband I made the big decision to leave my teaching job to focus on my entertainment career, not even really thinking about the life coaching aspect. What I didn't realize at the time, is that it would give me the space to connect with my truest self and find my absolute passion and purpose, thus making me an even better, more confident mom and woman.

I gave notice at my job, and left when Noella was eighteen months old, feeling sad to leave my job helping children. I liked it a lot, and it was very meaningful, but a freedom to be with my baby and family and truly follow my passions was emerging. I had time. I had space. I had more balance. I started to read, attend a lot of workshops and seminars, spend time with my baby, and basically search. I knew I was open to finding my purpose and passions. I also knew the space was what I needed to find it.

I began praying and asking for my perfect self-expression. I knew that if I was to figure it out, it would help me be a happier,

By Betsy Chasse and Debbie Spector Weisman

better, more fulfilled mother, and live by example for my daughter to also be in her own power, purpose and confidence. I reminded myself regularly that a happy mommy means a happy baby, and a confident mom means a calm child.

Fortunately, I now had time to implement meaningful mommy baby bonding activities such as yoga, her first art class, and even baby tumbling with Tumble N' Kids, an extraordinary gymnastics company in Southern California. I took her grocery shopping with ease, to the car wash and even to doctor visits without the prior anxiety and stress. My husband was also very interested in self-development and personal growth to grow and develop ourselves, but to also be excellent parents, and communicate better with our child. We began to attend seminars and workshops more often, even getting certified in Neuro Linguistic Programming, which helped both our communication as a couple, and with Noella. We began going on more trips as a family, and taking baby out to dinner and to events more often.

Magically and beautifully around the time that Noella was three, I realized that what I wanted to do full force was to be a life coach. With my degree, credentials, personal development background, and other certifications, I was already ready. I set out in the world with my business as a coach, and began getting clients immediately. This led to many experiences such as a Ted Talk, motivational and inspirational speaking, writing my #1 bestselling book *Getting Your Life to a Ten+*, and more. I was finally in my life's purpose and passion, and was able to feel fulfilled, peaceful, a great mom, and on fire about what I did.

Currently, I now have two girls who are six years apart and very best friends, am very happy with my husband, and have quite a good life balance. I am confident, happy and fulfilled to be doing what I am passionate about, for having a caring and amazing family, and for being fit and healthy and positive. I do have a great life, but that doesn't mean I don't have days where I am moody, impatient with my kids, have trouble getting focused with work, etc. Don't forget to keep working on you. I promise you that life can become extraordinary, but don't expect perfection. Part of being human is the trips, falls and emotions. Enjoy the scenery, adventure and the ride.

By Betsy Chasse and Debbie Spector Weisman

Here are some tools, tips and wisdom for stepping into success, balance, power and confidence easily and effortlessly as a woman and a mother in simple steps.

1. **Choices**: Make sure that you are aware of your choices. Choose with your heart where you will live, what you do for a living or for your life purpose and passions, be careful of whom you spend time with, and what you read, watch and do. Choose your attitude, habits and behaviors.

2. **Connectedness**: Have a strong connectedness with your truest self. You can achieve this through journaling, spending time in nature, breathing, meditating, doing yoga, and self-care. You also can learn about yourself by asking those you trust for feedback. Email eight people that you know, like and trust and ask them how they see you, what gifts and talents they see in you, and any constructive criticism they may have for you. This may be uncomfortable, but is a great way to see yourself as others see you.

3. **Connections:** (spend time with those who "S.U.E." you; support, uplift and encourage you), and you them. Do not waste your energy and time with those who create drama, complain or drag you down to their level. This is especially important as a mom, as you continuously bring that energy home to your children or babies.

4. **Consciousness:** Be aware of yourself, your sensations, emotions, surroundings and actions. Don't let yourself robotically and monotonously go through each day, but rather flow through it, being in the now, conscious of self, others and your environment and life.

5. **Communication**: Be aware of your communication. Instead of using words like stressed, overwhelmed and frustrated, use challenging self to be greater, in demand and fascinated.

6. **Creations:** Create your own opportunities and jump into them, sculpting your own life by design. Don't wait for life to

happen. Research, ask for help, follow your dreams, and do what you love. Regularly make a list and evaluate everything you are doing in your life now, and what you wish to be doing as your dreams and goals. Rate each on your list as 0-100%, zero being that you hate it, and 100 that it sets you on fire and you love it. The goal eventually will be to only do things that you are 100% about. This includes spending time with people, careers, taking on hobbies and projects, and more.

7. **Check In**: At least three times per day use the A through G checklist to be in tune with yourself and your life as a mom. Ask yourself: How is my attitude, behaviors, and my communication? Am I following my dreams? Am I enthusiastic and exuberant? How is my focus? Am I consistently growing as a person.

Parenting Thomas
By Kasia Wezowski

- A first time, new mom to Thomas 5 months old

My connection with Thomas started when I was pregnant. Long before I knew that he is a boy. I sneezed for the first time in the life of Thomas when I was four months pregnant, and I felt that he contracted his tiny body inside me. He was probably surprised and scared by this new sound. In the fifth month I started feeling his tiny legs and arms. When I went skiing I felt that after one hour on the slopes, Thomas started recognizing the movements of my body and imitating them. I felt his very tiny leg in my right side when I was turning right and in the left side of my belly when I was turning left. It seemed that he really liked skiing. He also started to make a rhythm with one of his hands when he was happy. He liked when I was eating strawberries, mango, Thai soup, and he also liked romantic music.

He was also able to distinguish when his father was close because he was putting his legs up in my belly creating a

By Betsy Chasse and Debbie Spector Weisman

'mountain' difficult to miss shape shown in my belly even for the father. Patryk was panicking a bit about our need to have a fulltime nanny and feared we'd end up with a baby who cried at all hours of the night. But I knew in my heart that he would be okay, that he would be sleeping well and be quiet, nice and joyful baby. This is how I felt him inside.

At the end of the pregnancy I loved to sleep with my baby and we slept till 9 or 10am and that two hours during the 'siesta' time. I trained him that when I was sleepy I starting breathing very slowly and relaxing my body. This was a signal for my baby to relax his body as well. He was also adjusting his body positions to my body.

In the ninth month I felt like a big whale turning from one side to the other in the bed. I was making some sounds and I experienced Thomas adjusting quickly to my new position so we were really hugging each other.

During my home birth I felt that he was really present with me and he started to make this happy rhythm when my contractions started getting stronger and I when to the bath with my midwife and Patryk. Then at the end of birth when his head was crowning, I felt his hand doing the rhythm again as if saying: Everything is all right with me, mama and I'm almost there with you. Maybe that's why he was born in a superman position with one of his arm before the head so my midwife had to help him to release the head.

After a few weeks of sleeping in the same bed with the newborn Thomas, when I finally overcame the fear that he would be waking up my hard-working husband with his crying, I adjusted my pillows well to really feel comfortable in bed with my breastfeeding baby. I realized that that he is a great silent happy baby. When he wanted to eat, he was just getting closer to me and starting putting his hands on me and tapping on my arm or kicking with his legs.

Everybody told us that we would be very tired all the time and we should sleep when the baby is sleeping, and we did just that. When Thomas was ten days into the 'siesta' time he went to sleep like a baby only can and we looked at each other and went to the swimming pool and to do other things. We just couldn't sleep so many hours as Thomas.

By Betsy Chasse and Debbie Spector Weisman

Thomas was also a 'kamikaze' when he was a newborn. He could slide down from any kind of pillow just by jumping out with his tiny body to get closer to me when he was hungry during the night. I don't know how those little bodies can move but he could move a yard in two seconds in his urge to eat and then start patting me with his hands and opening his mouth as much as he could.

At the beginning we had to both learn how to find the way from my nipple to his mouth and after the birth we were really exhausted. For the first days we were trying very hard--sometimes as long as five minutes--to get him latched to my breast. I was laying down on one side trying to come closer to Thomas in many possible ways and he was opening his mouth the best he could. Sometimes we fell asleep trying, but we'd try again 30 minutes later and finally succeed.

When Thomas was five-days-old, Patryk had to travel to Belgium for one day and stay there for a night. I still felt my muscles and bones after giving birth, and I didn't want to carry Thomas too much myself, especially since he was already a heavy healthy little boy who didn't lose any weight after the birth.

It Came Out of my Vagina! Now What?!

I had somebody to help me with the house during the day and to change diapers of Thomas but then I was alone from 5pm. This was the time that Thomas wanted to have a little walk in somebody's arms because he was bored to be laying with me all day and I didn't feel like walking so much with my still trembling hip bones. So when he started crying for his walk I put him in the stroley but he didn't like it. He wanted to walk in my arms and he cried even louder. I didn't want to walk with him because he was so heavy and I was still weak. I started singing to him. But that didn't work. He cried more that he wanted his walk. Finally I cried. That must have shocked him. He looked at me and immediately stopped crying. Till the end of the day and during the night he was a nice happy and quiet baby again.

Thomas doesn't mind my business calls and he doesn't mind that I'm in front of my laptop a lot. When he was born we arranged an arm chair for me with legs support and with many pillows. We also organized a table in front of me and a small table for food and water. Thomas is able to sleep on me and breastfeed on me and I can work.

By Betsy Chasse and Debbie Spector Weisman

When he started making his first sounds, he was sometimes making a funny sound in crucial moments of my conversation. I liked Thomas being part of the calls because I could never become too serious and stressed about any business topic. Thomas was always so cute that it was soaking my heart and this tenderness I felt was also helping my business calls to be more friendly and authentic.

Thomas adores joining me at my business meetings. Starting from the time he was two to three months old, he was entertained by watching new faces and hearing new voices. We also experienced that there is something special about business meetings with baby Thomas because people open their souls when they see Thomas smiling.

Because of Thomas, the purpose of making business changed a lot for me. Before I was making calls for rational reasons to grow our business. Now I listen to my intuition and if I don't feel the connection with somebody, I finish the call very quickly. I just feel that I want to have a positive energy around Thomas, so if I don't like somebody's personal energy, I don't talk with them. Many times in the first weeks after Thomas was born I was forgetting about my calls at all. I was over the moon, and money and all the freaking out busy urgent agendas didn't apply to me. I had to do everything with my own pace with Thomas, conserving our rhythm that we developed. I also discovered that I could create the availability in my agenda around my baby rhythm.

Patryk and I are more self-aware right now of the kind of people we would like to attract to be around us. Having business meetings with Thomas taught us that people have different personal energies and different hidden agendas that we don't need to be part of. With some people Thomas could spend time for hours on my lap, with some people he was becoming impatient and we respected Thomas' opinion in our business decision. Life is more fun if you can make business with your whole family.

Creating a family brought a new meaning to our life. I realized that as a mum, my physical presence is very important for a baby. During the first three months of Thomas' life all the babysitters we scheduled to support us and help with the baby where actually mostly doing the house work and the dishes so that I can stay more with him.

I stopped doing things around the house, in order to be with Thomas almost all the time and any activities I was doing, I was doing with Thomas. He was with other people not more than two hours a day so that I could spend some time with Patryk alone or take a shower.

I love that Thomas is part of what we do. He can stay very peaceful and patient during our webinars and coaching sessions. He was even on our TV show. He has a trick he does when he wants to be with me. He shows our nanny that he is very hungry and starts crying, which forces her to bring him to me. Many times, though, when he is finally with me, he doesn't eat or eats just a little. Then he smiles his big smile, happy to be with me again. We don't want him to cry, so he participates in our activities. He feels when something is an important activity for us and he doesn't want to miss it.

Thomas is very supportive when we have a presentation, training, coaching session or a webinar and he can stay quiet, silently observing what's going on. The only place I'm still having challenge taking him is yoga. When we go to practice yoga with a group, it means that he walks with a nanny and he never likes it. He cannot understand that mama is having fun without him. He wants to participate as well.

On the other hand, I can practice yoga at home and he loves that. He watched my legs and arms doing big movement with surprise and amazement. He loves my child pose. I put Thomas in his seat and do the child pose for a moment. Then I rise above him and he smiles so much. Then I repeat and do the child pose again. He waits in silence. Then I rise up again and he smiles with his squealing sound.

Creating a family also has a new meaning for Patryk. Before having children, I asked him once if he really wanted to have children. I was afraid that he didn't want to have children because he already has children from his first marriage. He likes being an entrepreneur and might think it a burden for him to take care of children. But he said that he wanted to have children with me, so we started planning a child when we moved to Spain. I was worried that I would not be able to work and that it would be hard to have a baby because of what I heard about babies crying and not sleeping when you want them. But I decided to have a baby anyway, even though I would need to take care of him or her all by myself.

I remember when we still lived in Belgium and we used to go for a walk around a lake in a park. In the spring there was a black duck preparing to conceive small duckies and sit on eggs. There was also her partner who was swimming around very quickly long distances to bring her sticks for her nests. She examined every stick carefully, using some and throwing the others away. He had a full time job finding suitable sticks for her.

I asked Patryk, "Will you bring me sticks when I get pregnant?" He smiled and said, "Yes". He brought me many sticks to our nest by working hard to find investors for our movie and planning the finances so that I didn't need to worry about it so much during my pregnancy, especially at the end when I needed to create a sacred space for my birth.

It Came Out of my Vagina! Now What?!

Midwife Madness and Flapjacks
By: Janet Swift

"It worked wonders for my Doberman", the lady in the health food store said as I picked the raspberry leaf tea from the shelf. Proudly five months' pregnant with my first child, you'd think nobody else had ever given birth! Foolishly, I was undeterred and completed my purchase because Sheila said it would aid delivery.

Sheila, our very mature antenatal class midwife said a lot of things, not least of which that the men should have a picnic packed in case THEY were hungry during the delivery. Oh Sheila, little did you know my husband would take you seriously when you suggested flapjacks would be essential pre-fatherly fodder and packed a snack bag just for himself, even disappearing for a lunch break although it was the middle of the night.

Oh boy, at 2.30am on 23rd January 1992, I thought it was 'mission go' as I awoke with pain. "Better have a shower and wash my hair before we leave for the hospital" I thought to myself. Husband decides he'll snooze for a while. Really?

By Betsy Chasse and Debbie Spector Weisman

Actually, I was a bit surprised as our 'son' wasn't due for another two weeks. But, hey, a girl has to follow Nature, right? Well, this girl should have ignored Sheila and her remedies. Oh, did I mention the lavender oil we were instructed to add to the bath water?

Excited but feeling a bit short changed as I should have had another two weeks of gliding around in full bloom, which I have to admit I loved, I focused on the moment. Life was about to change in such an irrevocable way. As a 35-year-old 'primagravida' – what a dreadful description of my happy condition - I'd taken a year's maternity leave to enjoy every moment of being a mother. Imagine my horror when our doctor said I'd have to be under the hospital consultant because "You're a very old lady for this sort of thing". (Years later, I reminded our doctor of this and he was horrified. "Did I really say that?" he asked. "I'm surprised you didn't have me struck off!" Hmmm, he certainly burst my bubble that afternoon.)

Husband finally dragged himself out of bed, I was freshly bathed and smelling like a flower meadow on a spring day and off we went. It was a thick frost and, as we approached the hospital, we noticed a massive building site where the Maternity Unit entrance used to be. Parking in the middle of said mess, husband asks if I'll be alright to make it to the door. Nope. Back in car and re-routed to the temporary door.

It was exciting in a frightening sort of way. The night nurse was kind if a little 'oh-God-not-another-one' and we were shown to a delivery room. We waited, and waited, and waited and were finally sent home as contractions weren't strong enough. Back out into the freezing early dawn I struggled, thankful the car was nearby. Home beckoned and some more raspberry leaf tea and a nice relaxing lavender oil infused bath seemed like a good idea.

It was a case of 'rinse and repeat' as we returned 24-hours later. Pain and lack of sleep had taken the edge off the enjoyment now and this time we were admitted to the ward. A young girl had a room of her own whereas we other 'expectants' shared a four-bedded bay. What I didn't know then was that the girl was about to deliver a stillborn child.

By Betsy Chasse and Debbie Spector Weisman

The day stretched ahead without much progress and a mobile ultrasound machine was brought to my bedside. Oh yes, baby was alive and well, sucking a thumb with one hand and tugging on the umbilical with the other! It so entertained the staff, others came to have a look. There'd been concern the delay was caused by insufficient fluid around the baby but he was just fine.

Finally, as they wanted the bed in the ward, we were shipped down to 'Delivery' and had a room to ourselves for the big moment. Only hours and hours passed with no progress, the midwife actually saying, "I'll be back in three hours" and left us to it – can you believe that? By now, I was falling asleep between contractions and the picnic and flapjacks had been consumed by husband in the day room. I labored on.

Now I know doctors work long hours but I was horrified when the same young woman came to me in the delivery room at 5am as I'd seen at 9am the day before! Long story short, having tried to put a cannula in my arm for the dreaded oxytocin drip to speed things up, she'd gone straight through the vein and, as my left arm started to inflate with fluid, she announces she's going to try on the other side. Raspberry leaf tea, why aren't you doing for me what you did for the Doberman delivery?

Next door, a Chinese lady wailed for hours, apparently to drive away evil spirits. In the distance, I heard my husband ask "is this nearly the end?" and I hoped he meant the delivery and not me! He touched my leg and as I said "Get Off", the midwife told me off! Me, the one in pain! "Don't you speak to him like that" she ordered. If I'd had the strength, I'd have flattened her but on gas and air and from my prone position, I decided to let it go. She's one very lucky lady, although I use the term loosely.

We were having a son, I was sure, because at the original ultrasound scan, I thought I saw the necessary bits and pieces and asked the radiographer who promptly turned the screen away. (In those days at our hospital they didn't divulge the sex of the baby.) Clearly, I was right and we were to be blessed with a boy. Everything I made was blue or lemon but deep down inside maybe I knew? I'd bought two blue and a pink cushion for the chair in the nursery.

By Betsy Chasse and Debbie Spector Weisman

At some point during labor, I'm sure all women think "I just don't want to do this anymore". As we drifted into a third day of labor, I went a thought further thinking death would be preferable. Tiredness takes its toll.

Eventually, at 6.21am on 25th January, a baby girl entered the world. A daughter. I was thrilled. Mind you, as she'd struggled so long to arrive, she looked like ET and had a strange blue hue. It was a minor miracle to see her color change and to see the bones of her head literally ping into place revealing a beautifully shaped head (so our home midwife later said) and to meet this little lady who'd journeyed long and hard to meet us. I loved her immediately and yet I wondered what to do next.

The first job was a bath but as I relaxed in the water, it turned a worrying shade of red. My only and immediate conclusion was that I must be bleeding to death. I pulled the emergency cord so I must have been worried, calling a complete stranger while I was in the bath. A big, happy West Indian woman arrived wearing a calming dark blue uniform. Thanks heavens, the Sister-in-Charge had answered my plea for help. "It's perfectly natural, nothing to worry about. I've had five children and I know you'll be fine". That's a relief then. I got out of the bath and went back into the delivery room for the 'embroidery'. Mentioning the 'emergency' to the sister doing my sewing, she revealed that the lady who'd come to advise me was in fact ... the cleaner! Really, how did that happen? Mind you, she did put my mind at rest and I didn't die.

Proudly cradling my baby daughter, a nurse pushed me in a wheelchair out of the delivery suite and my husband carried the bags, lighter now as he'd enjoyed a night's feasting between contractions. It's a girl, I merrily shared with everyone who smiled at me, making a mental note to self to send a "please send pink things" message when I could. Remember, this was long before the mobile phone made its debut. A nurse from the original ward was on her way home. "Oh there you are" she said, "You've been gone so long we thought you'd been transferred to another hospital".

As we neared the lift, we came upon our local surgery midwife, not Sheila of the flapjacks but Mavis, a stern-faced spinster. She didn't say "how wonderful that you've had a healthy baby" but floored me with, "now you've had the baby you can get some of that weight off". It wasn't just me taken aback but also the kind young nurse with us.

After a piece of toast and seeing the baby still asleep in her little fish tank-type crib, I finally drifted off to sleep after almost three days. I don't think falling asleep between contractions counts.

After just twenty minutes, I was startled awake. "Have you considered contraception going forward?" was the question which warranted snatching me from my slumber. *What? There will never be reason ever again to require contraception,* I thought. This is another very lucky lady because, had I had the strength, I think I'd have taken a swing at her, too. Why wake someone with such a stupid question? Apparently, they have to tick the box to say they've mentioned it. Don't worry, you won't be seeing me in Delivery *ever* again.

The next time I awoke, it was because a pair of blue eyes were watching me. My beautiful little girl was awake and quietly looking at me through the Perspex side of her crib. Oh my

It Came Out of my Vagina! Now What?!

goodness, what shall I do now? I gingerly picked up the little bundle and cuddled her to me. Still she didn't cry but looked inquisitively at me.

Over the next 24-hours, I was told never to wake a sleeping baby to feed it and, conversely, was asked why I hadn't woken my baby girl after four hours to feed her! Conflicting advice is so confusing to new mums, especially first-timers. Let common sense prevail at all times!

On Day 3, we were discharged and, upon looking at my notes noticed the problems had been attributed to "incompetent uterus". Sheila's raspberry leaf tea and lavender oil baths had hastened the birth by two weeks. Clearly my darling daughter just wasn't ready, as evidenced by the jaundice which soon developed.

What worked for the Doberman, didn't work for my daughter!

By Betsy Chasse and Debbie Spector Weisman

Motherhood's Not for Punks
by Patrina Wisdom

Creating and cultivating community.

When managing four kids and a business as a single mother, life moves very fast. I am always doing and creating, nurturing and taking care of people or things. And I do my best to stay in the moment because that's about as much as my mind can handle. I don't have the energy to dwell on yesterday or worry about tomorrow.

The exercise of writing and completing my book "Motherhood's not for Punks" has been such a gift because it reflected back to me my incredible journey. I have managed and moved through so much since losing my husband to suicide and finding out that I was pregnant with my fourth child the same day in 2009.

A little over 2 years ago (February 2013) I woke up with a knowing that it was time to leave Las Vegas. It was time to release all of my crutches, release the memories of life with my husband, release who I'd been and walk away from everything I knew to discover who I'm meant to be, and create my fresh start.

Twenty eight days later I packed up my four kids, sold my house and left Las Vegas where I had family, friends, and support to move to San Diego where I knew no one and nothing. My transition has been a wild and crazy and beautiful ride but it's also been a *really* hard one - a journey that I share more about in my book.

In two short years I've gone from knowing no one and having no support with my kids or my new business, and not knowing how to ask or receive help to cultivating a beautiful community of friends and mentors, learning how to ask and receive support and love, building an incredible brand, and preparing to publish my first book.

The days of woman being catty and in competition with each other are gone. It's an old played out paradigm that doesn't serve us as women. We live in an abundant Universe. There is plenty money, and men, and beauty to go around. The only way to grow stronger as women and as a community; the only way to move

By Betsy Chasse and Debbie Spector Weisman

humanity forward and raise incredible kids, is to realize that we are all reflections of each other. It takes a village to raise a child. It takes a village of beautiful reflections of yourself to remind you of your strength and your beauty in the moments when you forget.

One of the most valuable lessons I've learned as a single mother of four since packing up my kids and moving to San Diego where I had no family or friends, is just how important it is to create and cultivate community. When you've lived someplace for a long period of time and you have family and friends there, it's easy to take it all for granted. But after floating in and out of Las Vegas for my entire life, it was time for me to go. I needed a fresh start and I was willing to do whatever it took to get it. Even though it meant leaving the village that had been so supportive to me.

You have to have that kind of conviction when you really want something. You have to be willing to take risks and make sacrifices. There is no playing it safe. There is no staying inside your comfort zone. In order to have big change, big Transformation, and big rewards, you have to make big sacrifices.

It Came Out of my Vagina! Now What?!

So how do you connect with like-minded women and create community?

Here are some tips:

Tip #1: Know thyself. If you know who you are, and what your needs are, you can seek out like-minded people to spend time with. Remember that you are the 5% average of the people you spend the most time with, so choose wisely.

Tip #2: Secure reliable childcare. Using care.com or a babysitting/nanny service or direct referral. When meeting other moms you can offer to share your childcare provider and split costs or point her in the right direction. You can also take turns caring for each other's kids.

Tip #3: Introduce yourself to your neighbors. Make the first move. Don't wait for them to talk to you. Find out who has kids. Invite them over for drinks or dinner. Be open to building relationships with the people closest to you.

Tip #4: Get out and meet new people. Take advantage of the fact that you're the hot new face in town (or in the room). Choose one new place a week to check out and go alone if you have to. A confident woman can go anywhere alone. I find that I usually meet the most interesting people when I do. Meetup.com is a great resource for meeting people because you can search activities according to interests.

Tip #5: Be interested rather than interesting. Do your best to ask a lot of questions and learn as much as you can about the people your meeting. Most people are so used to everyone talking about themselves and what they do that there is no time or space for the other person to share. Flip it. Be genuinely interested in learning about them and then be open to share once they start asking you questions.

Tip #6: Be of service. One of the best ways to meet great people is to align with a charity or outreach group that resonates with you. What better way to meet like-minded, service oriented people?

Tip #7: Find your peeps and cultivate a sisterhood. We all need connection. No one wants to feel alone. Long periods of disconnection can cause you to feel depressed and it can diminish your self-esteem. Be proactive about aligning with other sisters to create circles of support, creation, and celebration.

Your community of support will not come to you. Someone has to initiate and create it. We all have obligations and demands on our time so connection and sisterhood often gets put on the back burner, but it's important and must be prioritized higher.

My sisters and I get together regularly to share our challenges, and support each other. We also spend a lot of time sharing our dreams and what we want to call in or create. Knowing and holding the intention for each other's dreams makes celebrating the accomplishment of the dreams that much more fun.

By Betsy Chasse and Debbie Spector Weisman

Chapter 20
The Final Word On Being a Mom

Betsy: Wow, you've made it all the way to the end of this book. Is your child still alive? Well good. Then guess what? You're probably an awesome mom.

That's basically the point of this entire book. You're going to be great, better than great. You're going to be fantasmic, amazeballs, brilliant! You're also going to screw up a lot, and chances are no matter what you do, as long as your kids feel loved, feel heard and respected as individuals, they are going to turn out just fine.

For too long we've been on the Halloween hayride to parenting hell, with books and guides and how to's, don't do's and should do's about parenting. We spend too much time worrying and not enough time just being with our kids, allowing them to find themselves when they want to and how they want to.

My big aha moment of realization that my kids were in fact individuals and not remote controlled extensions of myself came on the day my son admitted his favorite color wasn't orange. He was just saying that because he thought it would make me happy. He actually really liked purple and he asked, "Is that okay Mommy, that I'm different from you?" Another toughie was when my daughter, who has the most beautiful singing voice, stated she didn't want to sing in front of people, not now or ever. She said it with such conviction, and so far, four years later, she still means it. That was her, not me.

In those moments I am reminded that my job is to not attempt to recreate myself, but instead to honor and guide the beings in front of me. My role is to foster their dreams, to hold their hands--but not too tightly--to let them fall and skin their knees and to watch them fly on their own. This is what Conscious parenting is all about. Listening to your kids, trusting your heart and not allowing your fear to rule the day. Using no when it's needed and saying yes, often, and most importantly hugging when you want to scream and riding the scary roller coasters with them, even if it makes you want to vomit.

By Betsy Chasse and Debbie Spector Weisman

Every day I learn something from my kids; they are my greatest teachers. I am in awe of how they learn, how they dream and how they express. It's not always easy; instilling the fear of god would make for a much quieter house, but not a very fun, loving house. Yep, my house is loud, with music, with laughter, with upset and joy and everything in between, and I like it that way.

Debbie: Being the mother of two adult children has given me lots of time to reflect on my parenting life. As you can well imagine, being a parent doesn't stop when they hit adulthood, it's a lifelong role that will transform and metamorphosis as you all enter different phases of growth and development. In this book I've sorta of provided a cautionary tale of some of the things that can go wrong as you maneuver your way through the maze of your children's early years. My thought is that forewarned is forearmed; the more you know about what "shouldn't be" will guard you against making the same mistakes I did.

What I may have left out are the quiet joys that reside as wonderful memories for me and my children—the cross country trips in the RV, putting together jigsaw puzzles on the dining room table, Friday night tickle time, jumping contests in the pool, the homemade Mother's Day gifts, playing dress up with my daughter, helping her buy her first formal gown, listening to my son make up songs in the back seat of the car, watching him break a board with his hand at Tae Kwon Do. Those are the moments that I remember now and there are countless others that will bubble up in my consciousness from time to time. One of my favorite memories is cuddling in bed with my little girl on Thursday nights watching *The Cosby Show*. In light of recent developments, I now have to wonder if this resulted in some horrible psychological damage I'll have to live with for the rest of my life!

The point is that being a parent will be the toughest job you'll ever have. You'll get blamed for anything that ever goes wrong and never receive the credit you deserve for the things that go right. You'll know in your heart, though, that you've done the right thing when you provide unconditional love from the time you first set eyes on that delicious little baby until the day you breathe your last breath.

By Betsy Chasse and Debbie Spector Weisman

My final word…go forth and multiply!

About the Authors

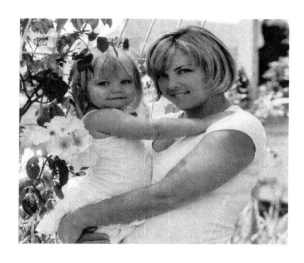

Betsy Chasse is mom to two children, Elora (11) and Max (8) and lives in Los Angeles, California. She is a film maker most notable for the break out documentary *What The Bleep Do We Know?!* and an author of four books, most recently *Tipping Sacred Cows*. She has been a featured writer on Huffington Post, Modern Mom and Intent.com and is a sought after speaker around the world on parenting, spirituality and filmmaking. She is currently in production on a new feature documentary about the world of life, relationship, business and executive coaching.

You can find out more about her at www.betsychasse.net

By Betsy Chasse and Debbie Spector Weisman

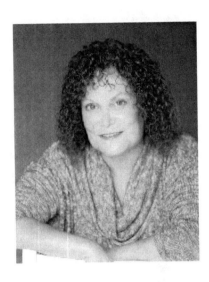

Debbie Spector Weisman has two adult children, a grandchild, and has been married for longer than she'd care to admit. Currently into her third career as a Dream-Life coach, Debbie is also co-owner of a company instrumental in the production of dozens of films including *What the Bleep Do We Know!?*, *Man of the Year*, starring John Ritter, and *Pregnant in America*. Debbie is also the best-selling author of over twenty novels, including five of the original books in the popular *Sweet Valley High* series. Her most recent book is *101 Dream Dates: How to Say I Love You To the Most Important Person in Your Life--You!* and is featured in *Chicken Soup for the Soul: Dreams and Premonitions* and *My Creative Thoughts*.

You can learn more about her at www.thedreamcoach.net

Contributing Authors

Kim Somers

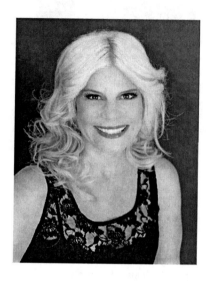

Kim Somers Egelsee is the #1 bestselling author of *Getting your Life to a Ten+*, a co-author of eight books, multi award winning Tedx and motivational speaker, life and business coach and confidence expert. She lives in Huntington Beach with her amazing husband and two daughters.

By Betsy Chasse and Debbie Spector Weisman

Kate Gardner

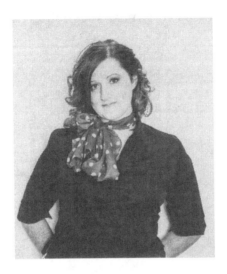

Kate Gardner is a 10 x International Best-Selling Author, Podcast Host, International Success Coach & CEO of The Missing Piece Publishing House.

As a Success Coach, Kate informs, motivates and empowers online business owners and helps provide them with the business tools and skills they need to succeed in their online businesses. Kate helps raise her client's self-esteem and self-confidence through providing tools to change their mind-sets so they are prepared for the responsibility that success brings to them.

As a publisher, Kate is the creator of the International Best Selling Book Series *The Missing Piece* which provides a platform for authors and online business owners to grow their network; with every intention of making them a best-selling author.

Kate's ultimate goal is to help you build a successful international platform and succeed in turning your followers into raving fans that constantly buy from you.

www.themissingpiecepublishing.com

www.the-missing-piece.net

By Betsy Chasse and Debbie Spector Weisman

Tanya Lynn

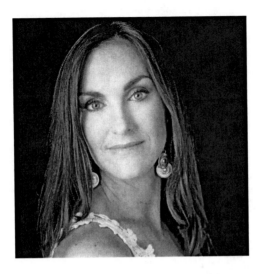

Tanya Lynn is the author of *Open Your Heart: How to be a New Generation Feminine Leader* where she vulnerably shares her own story to inspire and give other women permission to step into their power. She is most passionate about training women how to lead women's circles in their local communities to develop sisterhood and feminine leadership. Tanya lives in Carlsbad CA with her husband Brent and daughter Kali. For more information go to sistershipcircle.com and tribal-truth.com.

It Came Out of my Vagina! Now What?!

Kevra Cherne

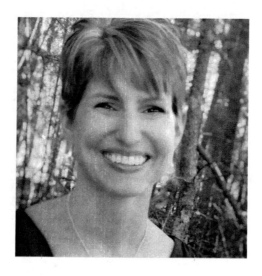

Kevra Cherne is straight-shooting accountant and business strategist who lives in Minnesota with her husband, three dogs and six children. She's been in business for the past ten years for herself and in the financial arena for nearly twenty. When she's not meal planning, helping clients make strategic plans for their business or taking the dogs out to pee she loves to eat, sleep and read (not necessarily in that order).

www.kevracherne.com

Patrina Wisdom

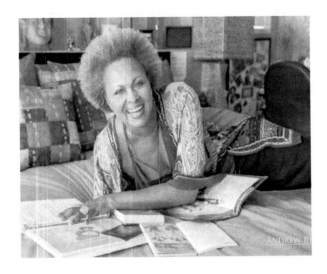

After losing her husband of 20 years to suicide and learning that she was pregnant with her fourth child the same day, Patrina Wisdom took two decades of experience as an entrepreneur and business leader, and began the process of her Badass Bodacious Life.

Fast forward 6 short years, She is a thriving CEO mom-preneur, published author, and a dynamic speaker that has graced the stages of Lisa Nichols, eWomen Network and TedX just to name a few… Find out more at www.patrinawisdom.com

It Came Out of my Vagina! Now What?!

Kasia Wezowski

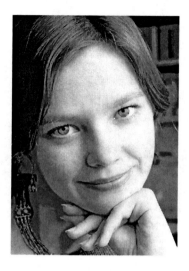

Kasia Wezowski is the producer of "Coaching", the first documentary about the coaching profession, the founder of the Center for Body Language, a creator of the Emotional Management Method and Micro Expressions Training Videos (METV). She is a unique Business Coach with 12 years' experience (with over 3000 coaching hours), and the creator of more than 30 methods for stress management, emotional consciousness and leadership development. She is an author of 4 best-selling books, appears in international media, including CBS, Fox, Forbes, at TEDx, in the full feature documentary Destressed and at Harvard University. Kasia has completed 3 university Master degrees at the same time: Psychology, Sociology and Law.

By Betsy Chasse and Debbie Spector Weisman

She is passionate about organizational dynamics, radical effectiveness without effort, intuitive creativity and human behavior. Combined with her passion for extreme traveling, immersing herself in exotic cultures, she believes that successful people normally do what the others do only sometimes. She is a mom of 5 months old Thomas who participates in all her activities from business calls to making movies.

It Came Out of my Vagina! Now What?!

Janet Swift

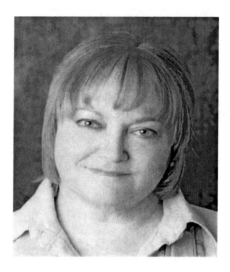

For 50 years Janet Swift accumulated every experience life could offer, seeking fulfilment through careers from nursing, police officer, 20+ years in the corporate world and finally, as a successful business owner. Despite this, she felt a burning sense of underachievement, recognizing her latent potential but, still believing it wasn't safe to shine her light, allowed her childhood decision to 'play small' to inform her next five decades, until life's hobnail boot startled her awake.

Janet's unique early life experience set her apart and the bright, intelligent expression of her truth was dimmed to survive as a seven-year-old child at boarding school. Raised in Bahrain, Malta and Germany herself, she's ensured her children are global citizens, encouraging them to pursue their dreams.

By Betsy Chasse and Debbie Spector Weisman

Now a #1 international bestselling author and coach, Janet shares her extensive knowledge and experience with her clients. Perhaps her greatest gift is enabling people from all walks of life to identify the events that have changed and shaped their choices and her range of workshops, talks and books are designed to captivate, inspire and encourage everyone to live their life on purpose and express their truth.

Are you living your dream or someone else's?

www.janetswift.com

It Came Out of my Vagina! Now What?!

Marla Keller

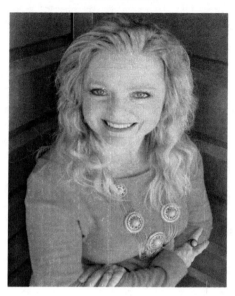

Marla became a mother in 1990 at the age of 21 and again at 22, and decided to put a hold on her university degree to raise her kids. When her girls went to school she enrolled in an Adult Degree Program at Greenwhich University, and in 2001, Marla finished her BA degree in Family Counseling. Marla, along with her husband of 27 years Jami, began their Relationship Coaching business part-time and volunteer in 1995 when they were Coach and Facilitator Certified with Life Skills International, and it has turned into a full-time career.

In 2009, Marla became Executive Coach Certified through **Invite Professional Coach Training**, and in 2011 turned Passion Provokers into a full-time job. They have been empty-nesters since 2013, and enjoy a connected relationship with their daughters, and their son-in-law of 3 years.

For more information please visit: www.passionprovokers.com/

By Betsy Chasse and Debbie Spector Weisman

Angela Mose

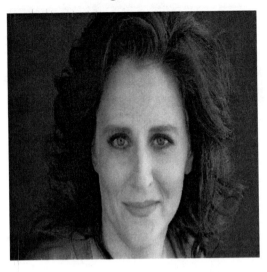

Angela Mosley is the Passionate Editor. She is also an Author and Ghostwriter. Angela believes that every person has a unique story to tell and that every story needs to be told. In her own story, Angela is Momma to three little ones--two boys code named Thing 1 and Thing 2, now 6 and 4 years old (born just 15 months apart—SURPRISE!), and Miss Pretty Pretty, now 2 years old. Her days are full of food drama and words…lots and lots of words, mostly all proceeded by the word "Why….." or followed by the words "Not fair!"

Website: www.angelamosley.com

Email: angela@angelamosley.com

Facebook: AngelaMosleyEditor

Twitter: @angelahmosle

It Came Out of my Vagina! Now What?!

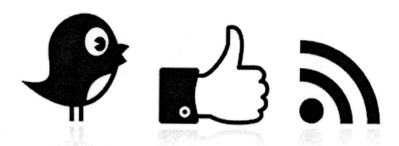

To find out more about Betsy Chasse go to **betsychasse.net**
To find out more about Debbie Spector Weisman go to **thedreamcoach.net**

Follow Betsy on Facebook, Twitter and Instagram **@betsychasse**
Follow Debbie on Facebook and Twitter **@dreamwithdebbie** and on Instagram **@thedreamcoach**

By Betsy Chasse and Debbie Spector Weisman

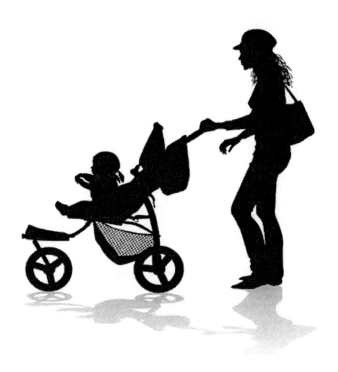

The End

CPSIA information can be obtained
at www.ICGtesting.com
Printed in the USA
FSOW01n1710180116
15673FS

9 781513 606750